Armed Forces Institute

MW01078698

Laboratory
Methods
in
Histotechnology

Edited by
Edna B. Prophet
Bob Mills
Jacquelyn B. Arrington
Leslie H. Sobin, M. D.

Prepared by the
Armed Forces Institute of Pathology
Washington, D.C.

Published by the
American Registry of Pathology
Washington, D.C.

Available from
American Registry of Pathology
Armed Forces Institute of Pathology
Washington, D.C. 20306-6000
ISBN:1-881041-00-X
1992

❖ CONTENTS

All authors were on the staff of the Armed Forces Institute of Pathology during the preparation of this book.

AFIP Laboratory Methods in Histotechnology

Introduction

High quality histopathology depends on high quality histotechnology. Microscope specimens that are substandard, i.e., poorly fixed, cut, or stained, impede the pathologist in making an accurate diagnostic evaluation.

The Armed Forces Institute of Pathology has long been concerned with promoting high standards of histotechnology, e.g., through its courses, publications, the Tri-Service Histopathology School, and its diagnostic consultative mission. This manual is an effort towards that goal.

In 1953, the late Mary Frances Gridley compiled the Laboratory Manual of Special Staining Techniques.[1] It was the outgrowth of notes that she first wrote by hand, then mimeographed. The manual comprised procedures Miss Gridley and her associates and predecessors in the laboratories at the AFIP found to be reliable and practical. A revised edition of this manual was published in 1957 as a memorial to Miss Gridley, who died in 1955. The title was changed to Manual of Histologic and Special Staining Techniques.[2] Financial support for its publication was obtained from various local and national societies interested in pathology and from the National Cancer Institute. The modifications and innovations in this revision were clearly the products of many members of the histopathology laboratory staff. In 1960, a second edition of the manual was printed by McGraw-Hill, New York.[3] In 1968, a third edition was produced as the Manual of Histologic Staining Methods of the AFIP, edited by Lee G. Luna.[4]

Dr. Robert F. Karnei, Jr., Director of AFIP from 1987 to 1991, recognizing the need to again update this manual to include new and current staining methods, initiated the revision process, and Dr. J. Thomas Stocker, Deputy Director, Army, guided the project through its many stages to completion, the resultant **AFIP Laboratory Methods in Histotechnology**. The authors wish to acknowledge Dr. Frank B. Johnson, Chief, Chemical Pathology, who provided valuable technical contributions; Ruth Tharrington and JoAnn Mills, for their expert assistance in editing the manuscript; and Fran Card, for originality in format design and preparation of the camera-ready copy.

The purpose of the current manual is to present the methods of histotechnology currently used at the Institute. It therefore approaches the subject from a practical rather than a theoretical viewpoint. Furthermore, it is written by those who perform the procedures on a daily basis. Consequently, it incorporates a number of modifications to published staining procedures that have been introduced over the years and provides useful advice on embedding, cutting, and processing. It is generally difficult to determine who actually introduced a specific modification. Thus, no attempt has been made to attribute such contributions to individuals. Suffice it to say that the Institute appreciates them and recognizes their importance in the evolution of histotechnological methods.

In this vein, the authors and editors welcome any comments or suggestions that will lead to the improvement of these procedures.

REFERENCES

[1]Gridley M F. *Laboratory Manual of Special Staining Techniques*. Washington, DC: Armed Forces Institute of Pathology; 1953.

[2]*Manual of Histologic and Special Staining Techniques*. Washington, DC: Armed Forces Institute of Pathology; 1957.

[3]*Manual of Histologic and Special Staining Techniques*. 2nd ed. New York, NY: McGraw-Hill; 1960.

[4]Luna LG, ed. *Manual of Histologic Staining Methods of the Armed Forces Institute of Pathology*. 3rd ed. New York, NY: McGraw-Hill; 1968.

❖ **CHAPTER 1**

LABORATORY SAFETY

Melvin W. Lynch, Jr.

Safety is fundamental to laboratory management and operation. The laboratory technician must be constantly aware of the hazards which are present and cognizant of how to overcome them.

Provided here is a basic plan to establish and update laboratory safety programs. Although histologic techniques are generally consistent from one laboratory to another, safety demands and requirements vary.

GENERAL STATEMENT ON LABORATORY SAFETY

A comfortable and safe environment provides a feeling of security and reduces apprehension about handling specimens, reagents, or equipment. Safety should be the primary concern of everyone in the laboratory. Many steps in histologic processing present some hazard or potential hazard. Everyone from the chief technician to the most recently hired employee should be made aware of the hazards and how to avoid them. Orientation, periodic briefings, review of standard operating procedures, laboratory safety manuals, and continuing education enhance awareness and the level of expertise within the laboratory.

STANDARD OPERATING PROCEDURES AND SAFETY MANUALS

All functions of a laboratory should be written concisely in the form of standard operating procedures (SOPs), including all phases of safety. SOPs should address every procedure, chemical, and piece of equipment within the laboratory. Electrical safety, infection control, first aid, accident reporting, inspections, and training should be included. The facility should produce a safety manual covering specific safety requirements and directions for each unit. The manual should be based upon guidelines established by the state and local governments and the requirements of the Occupational Safety and Health Administration (OSHA), National Institute for Occupational Safety and Health (NIOSH), Joint Commission on Accreditation of Hospitals, College of American Pathologists, and other relevant organizations. Safety manuals and SOPs are the cornerstones of the safety program.

SAFETY TRAINING

Having SOPs and safety manuals will not prevent accidents. To have an effective safety program everyone must be made aware of how to respond or react in any particular situation. Safety training should be a part of the initial briefing, regardless of the level of experience of the employee. Periodic briefings (at least monthly) must be given to all employees. These safety briefings should be informative, up to date, and relevant. Updated safety briefings should accompany the introduction of new procedures, chemicals, reagents, or infectious agents.

Accident reporting and response measures are emphasized to ensure that in the event of an accident appropriate action will be taken. Everyone must have confidence in the program and each other's ability to respond in case of an accident. The facility should provide periodic (at least annual) training in the areas of cardiopulmonary resuscitation, first aid, and firefighting for all employees. To ensure that employees receive the required training, all briefings, classes, and lectures must be documented for each employee. Training records must be accessible to the employees and their immediate supervisors and must be kept up to date.

WARNING SIGNS AND LABELS

Warning signs and labels should be pointed out and explained to the new employee. All reagents and chemicals must be labeled to show date opened or made, by whom made, expected shelf life, and any precautions to be observed. Many companies now provide safety data sheets with each chemical. These should be kept available for reference. National Fire Prevention Agency labels are also available to provide information on chemicals and reagents. All refrigerators and freezers must have signs to show their contents, restrictions, and limitations. Within each laboratory a highly visible, easily accessible safety bulletin board should be available to post needed information on accident reporting forms and procedures, current handling procedures for chemicals and specimens, and important telephone numbers. All emergency equipment and facilities, including deluge showers, eyewash stations, fire extinguishers, fire blankets, first aid kits, spill kits, broken glass disposal locations, and hazardous chemical disposal locations, should be labeled to specifically identify their use. Additionally, each laboratory exit should have posted on or near it an emergency evacuation route.

PROTECTIVE CLOTHING AND FIRST AID

A safe work place contains safety equipment and protective clothing to reduce the possibility of accidents, injuries, or infection. Among the necessary items are protective gloves; aprons and face shields or goggles for use with toxic or hazardous chemicals; and surgical gloves, masks, surgical gowns, and head and foot coverings for use with hazardous specimens. Laboratory coats or other protective garments should be worn at all times while working in the laboratory. They should not be worn outside the laboratory if there is risk of spreading contaminants. A list of safety items appears in Table 1 -1.

One of the most important items is a fully stocked First Aid Kit. All personnel should be trained in first aid and have a ready access to the location and phone number of a medical response team, medical facility, and/or physician.

HANDLING OF HAZARDOUS CHEMICALS

Many chemicals are used in the laboratory, and each presents health hazards and storage requirements which must be addressed. It is the responsibility of both supervisor and technician to be familiar with current requirements for the safe handling of chemicals.

Right to Know laws require that Material Safety Data Sheets (MSDS) for each chemical in use be readily accessible to all personnel. There are numerous manuals, pamphlets, and regulations available which can assist or direct technologists in the proper method of handling and storing of chemicals. Some of these manuals are available free of charge through local, state, or federal government agencies. The NIOSH Pocket Guide to Chemical Hazards, published by the U.S. Department of Health and Human Services, can be purchased from the Superintendent of Documents, U.S. Government Printing Office, Washington, D.C. 20402.

The use of protective clothing and equipment when handling hazardous chemicals is mandatory. Placing containers in their proper location and keeping the work area neat and organized will greatly reduce accidental spills and breakages.

In the event of a chemical spill, all personnel in the area should be notified and if evacuation of the laboratory is necessary, their exit must be immediate. The correct spill kit should be used and the appropriate individuals and agencies notified.

In order to prevent explosions when decanting flammable liquids, it is necessary to ground metal containers. This can be accomplished by attaching an alligator clip to a piece of wire which is securely attached to a metallic water pipe. When pouring the liquid from one container to another, the clip should be attached to the container into which the liquid is being poured; this will help prevent static electricity from producing a spark, which could result in an explosion.

DISPOSAL OF HAZARDOUS CHEMICALS

For the proper disposal of hazardous chemicals the local or state government is the regulating agency. Guidelines established by these agencies are disseminated to all user organizations and should be available within each laboratory. Safety officers and fire marshals should be able to assist with questions and provide guidance. A central repository area is required which is used for holding the waste until it can be picked up by a disposal company. The laboratory is responsible for segregating the waste by type; labeling the containers as to content, date, and name of laboratory; naming the responsible individual to contact; and listing the hazards present in transporting the waste containers from the laboratory to the pickup or holding point.

The method of disposal (incineration, dilution, flushing down the drainage system, recycling, autoclaving, or transfer to landfills) will depend upon the type of chemical.

STORAGE OF FLAMMABLES

As a general guideline it is recommended that the quantity of flammable and combustible reagents kept in the laboratory not exceed that used daily. When flammable liquids are kept within approved safety containers the total capacity allowed within the laboratory should not exceed 60 gallons per 5,000 square feet. A minimum of one approved flammable storage room should be available if the reserve storage required is in excess of 300 gallons.

Flammables should not be stored within 18 inches of electric lights, steam pipes, sprinkler heads, and ceilings. Items which are susceptible to water damage should be stored on skids or pallets at least 4 to 12 inches off the floor, the exact distance depending on flood conditions of the area.

Flammables should be stored in approved metal containers which can be ventilated. Refrigerated flammables must be stored in explosion-proof refrigerators. Each container is placed in a position which is easily accessible and as low as possible to the floor. A safety cabinet should never be placed above eye level, where it is necessary to reach overhead to obtain the chemicals. These cabinets should be labeled as to contents and hazards.

SAFETY INSPECTIONS

Safety inspections are a means of ensuring that prescribed guidelines are followed and serve to reveal potential hazards.

Any formal inspection by extramural authorities includes a thorough review of safety procedures, equipment, and work practices within the laboratory. Documentation must be available to show that procedures are followed and to verify that required training has been provided. Records must show who received the training, when it was conducted, and who presented it. Preventive maintenance records, which document proper functions of safety equipment, must be available for review.

In addition to formal inspections by outside agencies, internal inspections must be conducted. These are scheduled at set intervals by the safety officer of the facility. In order to provide consistency in these internal inspections a list of questions should be answered each time. These questions, in the form of a checklist, should be periodically reviewed and updated if necessary. After completion of the checklist by the inspector, a copy is kept in the laboratory along with a copy of the responses to any discrepancy found. An example of such a checklist (AFIP General Safety Inspection Checklist) is presented as Table 1-2.

MICROWAVE HISTOTECHNOLOGY
Frank B. Johnson

The application of microwaves is emerging as a valuable adjunct in histotechnology. Various authors have recommended its use in all of the usual steps of tissue processing for paraffin or plastic sectioning and for a wide variety of histologic and histochemical stains. Although we have found the microwave oven useful for rapidly prewarming solutions to 56°C it has not been suitable for the large volume of histologic material in our laboratories. In any event, it is important to recognize the following safety precautions.
1. Food items must not be heated in the oven used for histotechnology.
2. The user must be familiar with the oven.
3. No sealed containers are to be used in the oven.
4. No metallic objects except the temperature probe are to be used in the oven.
5. No flammable or explosive substances are to be heated in the oven. These include alcohols and most usual clearing agents.

Almost any commercially available microwave oven is suitable for microwave histotechnology. The following characteristics are desirable.
1. An output of 500 or more watts.
2. Temperature probe reading from 90-200°F.
3. Provision for temperature hold.
4. Time control to nearest second.
5. Provision for rotating microwave beam or heating container.

Table 1-1

SAFETY EQUIPMENT AND PROTECTIVE GEAR

EQUIPMENT
    FLAME CABINET(S)
    MICROTOME KNIFE GUARDS
    RESPIRATOR
    EXPLOSION-PROOF REFRIGERATOR
    SAFETY SHOWERS
    EYEWASH STATION
    FUME HOOD
    SPILL KITS (with instructions)
    FIRE EXTINGUISHERS
    FIRE BLANKETS
    GROUNDED ALLIGATOR CLIPS
    GLASS DISPOSAL BOX
    FIRST AID KIT
    EMERGENCY LIGHTING
    ACID CARRIERS
    MECHANICAL PIPETTER
    SANDBOX
    EAR PROTECTORS
    3-PRONG ELECTRICAL PLUGS
    ANTISYPHON SINK DEVICES
    "LIPPED" SHELVES

PERSONAL PROTECTIVE GEAR
    GLOVES (Surgical, Rubber, Insulated)
    BOOTS (Surgical, Rubber overshoes)
    FACE SHIELDS
    SAFETY GLASSES
    SURGICAL MASKS
    SURGICAL SUITS
    SURGICAL GOWNS
    APRONS (Surgical, Rubber, Lead [X-ray])
    LAB COATS

TOXIC-FREE WORK AREA

The above represents a partial list of equipment and protective wear common to most histopathology laboratories. The list should be considered basic. Additional items may be required to meet the specific needs of a laboratory and its personnel.

Table 1-2

AFIP GENERAL SAFETY INSPECTION CHECKLIST

1. Is a list of hazardous chemicals and of explosive, toxic, carcinogenic or suspected carcinogenic compounds available in each laboratory?

2. Are all containers of hazardous materials labeled clearly to indicate the content?

3. Are all empty containers used for wastes labeled to indicate the name of the laboratory or source?

4. Do all cabinets containing hazardous materials have proper and conspicuous labels which warn users of the hazards?

5. Has each employee received complete written instructions for the safe handling, first aid, and decontamination procedures for each of the hazardous chemicals in the laboratory?

6. Do supervisors instruct each employee concerning safety procedures and is there documentation of the dates of the instruction?

7. Are all flammable and hazardous chemicals stored in approved safety cabinets?

8. Is personal protective gear available and used?

9. Are deluge showers available for each laboratory area and are they tested and tagged annually?

10. Are NO SMOKING signs posted in all laboratories?

11. Are all fire extinguishers and fire blankets mounted and within easy reach?

12. Does the emergency lighting system work and indicate when it was tested?

13. Is food stored in refrigerators which contain chemicals, solutions, and tissue specimens?

14. Are all damaged and torn floor and ceiling tiles replaced?

15. Do sinks with hoses attached to potable water plumbing fixtures in the laboratories, housekeeping utility closets, and other areas have vacuum breakers installed?

16. Do records of the quality checks of the water indicate the corrective action to be taken when the tolerance limits are exceeded?

❖ CHAPTER 2

LABORATORY CALCULATIONS

Jacquelyn B. Arrington

PERCENT SOLUTIONS
Volume/Volume

Percent solutions are prepared based on parts per 100 ml of the solvent. Percent may be expressed as parts per 100, whole number percents, or as a 2-place decimal. For example, eight percent can be expressed as 8/100, 8%, or the decimal equivalent 0.08. To convert a percent to a decimal, always move the decimal point (which is understood to be in the same position as the percent sign) two places to the left.

$$1\% = 01\% = 0.01$$

To prepare 200 ml of a 1% solution of acetic acid, first convert the 1% to a decimal as illustrated above. Multiply the final volume required (200 ml) by the decimal to obtain the amount of acid needed to make the diluted solution:

$$
\begin{array}{rl}
200 \text{ ml} & = \text{final volume} \\
\underline{X\ 0.01\quad} & = \text{required percentage} \\
2.00\ \text{ml} & = \text{amount of concentrated acid}
\end{array}
$$

Add 2 ml of concentrated acetic acid to 198 ml of distilled water to obtain 200 ml of a 1% solution.

Weight/Volume

For dry, crystalline, or powdered chemicals percentages are based on weight to volume. A 1% solution is 1 gm of the chemical per 100 ml of solution and can be calculated as described above.

To prepare 100 ml of a 5% borax solution:

$$
\begin{array}{rl}
100\ \text{ml} & \text{final volume} \\
\underline{X\ 0.05\quad} & \text{required percentage} \\
5.00\ \text{gm} & \text{of borax needed}
\end{array}
$$

Weigh 5 gm of borax and add distilled water in a quantity sufficient to bring the final volume to 100 ml.

Dilutions

It is often necessary to dilute solutions that are not 100% concentrations, e.g., the preparation of 70% alcohol for the Gridley fungus stain or for use on the tissue processor from 95% stock alcohol.

The formula is: $$V_1 \times C_1 = V_2 \times C_2,$$
where V_1 is the unknown quantity we are solving for, C_1 is the concentration of the stock solution, V_2 is the final volume we require, and C_2 is the diluted concentration we want to prepare.

To prepare 300 ml of 70% alcohol from a 95% stock alcohol solution:

$$V_1 \times C_1 = V_2 \times C_2$$
$$V_1 \times 95 = 300 \times 70$$

$$V_1 \times 95 = 21000$$
$$V_1 = 21000/95$$
$$V_1 = 221 \text{ ml (rounded)}$$

To 221 ml of 95% alcohol add 79 ml of distilled water to obtain 300 ml of a 70% alcohol solution.

Be sure that the units used for each volume and for each concentration are the same on both sides of the equation.

Dilutions as Ratios

Some formulas state dilutions as a ratio such as 1:2 or 1:4.
A 1:4 ratio may be expressed as one part in a total of 4 parts. To dilute stock Fontana silver solution for a 1:4 working solution:

Required volume = 100 ml;
100 ml /4 = 25 ml (each of the 4 parts is 25 ml);
1 part stock solution = 25 ml
+ 3 parts distilled water = 75 ml
4 parts (required volume) = 100 ml.

DYE CONTENT

The actual percentage of contained dye may vary significantly from dye lot to dye lot or from manufacturer to manufacturer. It may become necessary to use more or less dye in solution preparation to correct for the varying dye concentration. If the percentage of actual dye content is provided by the manufacturer, a ratio may be used to correct the weight of the dye required; if the percentage is not provided, experimentation with the new dye lot will be required. If a dye solution is staining correctly at 1 gm per 250 ml and the dye has a dye content of 78%, a new dye lot with a dye content of 62% may not produce adequate results at the same concentration. The solution may be corrected as follows:

(1) old dye content divided by new dye content = correction ratio
78/62 = 1.26;
(2) old weight times the correction ratio = new weight
1 gm X 1.26 = 1.26 gm.
Use 1.26 gm of dye for each 250 ml of dye solution.

MOLAR SOLUTIONS

Molar solutions prepared from solid materials are defined as one gram molecular weight of the substance dissolved in 1000 ml of the solvent. Find the molecular weight of the substance using a periodic chart, or it may be listed on the chemical container.

To prepare 500 ml of a 1.5 molar solution of sodium hydroxide, we perform the following calculations:

(1) Find the molecular weight of sodium hydroxide (NaOH):
sodium (Na) = 22.98 (from the periodic chart)
oxygen (O) = 15.99
hydrogen (H) = 1.01
_____
molecular wt = 39.98

A one molar solution of NaOH contains 39.98 gm of NaOH per 1000 ml of water.

(2) Gram molecular weight X molarity X volume in liters

39.98 grams X 1.5 Mole X 0.5 L = 29.98 gm
Slowly add 29.98gm of NaOH to enough water to bring the final solution volume to 500 ml.

Note. If the units of measure illustrated above are used (gram molecular weight, molarity expressed as a decimal, and volume in liters expressed as a decimal), a simple multiplication formula is all that is required and no cross multiplication or divisions are necessary. Be sure that you express the units of measure as demonstrated.

Dilution Factors for Liquids

In addition to the above formula, calculations for molarity of liquids such as some acids and bases require the use of a dilution factor based on the actual concentration of the substance and the specific gravity of the substance.

To prepare 200 ml of 0.5 molar hydrochloric acid we perform the following calculations:

HCl has a gram molecular weight of 36.5.

(1) 36.5 gm X 0.5 Mole X 0.2 L = 3.65 gm

Each milliliter of hydrochloric acid weighs 1.19 gm (specific gravity), and pure hydrochloric acid accounts for 37% of the 1.19 gm (concentration as provided by the manufacturer). To find the dilution factor;

(2) specific gravity X concentration (as a decimal)

1 .19 X 0.37 = 0.44
3.65 gm /0.44 = 8.3 ml

To 191.7 ml of water slowly add 8.3 ml of HCl to obtain 200 ml of a 0.5 molar solution.

Remember, as a safety precaution always add acid slowly to the water. Never add water to concentrated acids.

NORMAL SOLUTIONS

A normal solution is defined as one gram equivalent weight of solute dissolved in one liter of solution. The gram equivalent weight is the quantity of a substance that will replace or react with 1.008 gm of hydrogen and is calculated by dividing the molecular weight of the substance by the number of replaceable hydrogen molecules (total oxidation number of cations or anions).

Prepare 3 liters of a 0.5 normal solution of sulfuric acid (H_2SO_4).

molecular weight = 98
specific gravity = 1.84
% of pure sulfuric acid per gram = 98%
# of replaceable hydrogens = 2

Gram equivalent weight = molecular weight / replaceable hydrogens

98/2 = 49 gm

Required substance weight = gram equivalent weight X normality (expressed as a decimal) X volume (expressed in liters)

49 gm X 0.5 normal X 3 L = 73.5 gm required.

This is an acid; thus the dilution factor must be used.

Dilution factor = specific gravity X concentration of pure acid

1.84 X 0.98 = 1.8 gm

There are 1.8 gm of pure acid in each milliliter of stock acid solution.

Grams required / dilution factor = volume required.

73.5 gm /1.8 gm per ml = 40.8 ml

Slowly add 40.8 ml of concentrated H_2SO_4 to 2959.2 ml of water to obtain 3 L of a 0.5 normal acid solution.

CONVERTING TEMPERATURES

It may be necessary to convert temperature measurements or settings from one scale to the other.

Fahrenheit = (Celsius X 9/5) + 32 or

Fahrenheit = (Celsius X 1.8) + 32

Celsius = (Fahrenheit - 32) x 5/9 or

Celsius = (Fahrenheit - 32) x 0.556

Remember to perform the calculations inside the parenthesis first.

❖ CHAPTER 3

SOLUTION PREPARATION

Jacquelyn B. Arrington and Edna B. Prophet

ACETIC ACID SOLUTIONS
   0.2% — 0.2 ml glacial acetic acid in 99.8 ml distilled water.
   1% — 1 ml glacial acetic acid in 99 ml distilled water.
   3% — 3 ml glacial acetic acid in 97 ml distilled water.
   5% — 5 ml glacial acetic acid in 95 ml distilled water.
   12% — 12 ml glacial acetic acid in 88 ml distilled water.

ACETIC ACID, FORMALIN, see Formalin, acetic acid.

ACETONE-XYLENE SOLUTION — Equal parts of acetone and xylene.

ACID ALCOHOL SOLUTION, 1% — 1 ml hydrochloric acid in 99 ml of 70% ethyl alcohol.

ACID FUCHSIN SOLUTION, 1% aqueous — 1 gm acid fuchsin in 100 ml distilled water.

ACIDIFIED WATER SOLUTION — To 500 ml sterile water (irrigation) add enough 0.3% citric acid solution to bring pH to 4.0 or slightly higher.

ACIDULATED WATER — 1000 ml triple distilled water. Add enough 1% aqueous citric acid to bring water to pH 4.0.

ALCIAN BLUE (8GS) SOLUTION — 1 gm alcian blue, 8GS in 100 ml distilled water then add 1 ml glacial acetic acid.

ALCIAN BLUE (8GX) SOLUTION, pH 0.4 — 2.5 gm alcian blue, 8GX in 250 ml phosphate hydrochloric acid solution.

ALCIAN BLUE (8GX) SOLUTION, pH 1.0 — 1 gm alcian blue in 100 ml of 0. 1 N hydrochloric acid solution (10 ml of 1 N hydrochloric acid solution in 90 ml distilled water).

ALCIAN BLUE (8GX) SOLUTION, pH 2.5, 1% — 1 gm alcian blue, 8GX in 100 ml 3% acetic acid solution.

ALCOHOLIC FORMALIN, see Formalin, alcoholic.

ALDEHYDE FUCHSIN SOLUTION — 1 gm basic fuchsin, 200 ml 70% ethyl alcohol then add 2 ml concentrated hydrochloric acid and 2 ml paraldehyde. Let stand for 2 to 3 days.

ALDEHYDE THIONIN SOLUTION — (Ch. 14)

ALKALINE ALCOHOL SOLUTION — 1 ml 1% sodium hydroxide in 100 ml of 50% ethyl alcohol.

ALUMINUM SULFATE SOLUTION, 5% — 5 gm aluminum sulfate in 100 ml distilled water.

AMMONIACAL SILVER SOLUTIONS
    SNOOK'S (Ch. 17)
    GOMORI'S (Ch. 17)
    MANUEL'S (Ch. 17)
    WILDER'S (Ch. 17)

AMMONIA WATER — 2 to 4 ml 28% ammonium hydroxide in 800 ml to 1000 ml distilled water.

AMMONIUM HYDROXIDE SOLUTION, 1% — 1 ml 28% ammonium hydroxide in 99 ml distilled water.

AMMONIUM SULFATE SOLUTION, 5% — 5 gm ammonium sulfate in 100 ml distilled water.

ANILINE BLUE SOLUTIONS
    Masson's — 2.5 gm aniline blue, 100 ml distilled water, add 2 ml glacial acetic acid.
    Bodian's — 0.1 gm aniline blue, 2 gm oxalic acid, 2 gm phosphomolybdic acid in 300 ml distilled water.

AZURE II - EOSIN SOLUTION — (Ch. 21)

BASIC FUCHSIN SOLUTIONS
    0.25% — 0.25 gm basic fuchsin in 100 ml distilled water or 1 gm basic fuchsin in 400 ml distilled water.
    1% — 1 gm basic fuchsin in 100 ml distilled water.

BIEBRICH SCARLET, 1% SOLUTION — 1 gm Biebrich scarlet in 100 ml distilled water.

BIEBRICH SCARLET - ACID FUCHSIN SOLUTION — 90 ml 1% Biebrich scarlet solution, 10 ml 1% acid fuchsin and 1 ml glacial acetic acid.

BORAX SOLUTIONS
    5% — 5 gm borax in 100 ml distilled water.
    Borax buffer — 19 gm borax in 1000 ml distilled water.

BORIC ACID BUFFER — 12.4 gm boric acid in 1000 ml distilled water.

BOUIN'S FIXATIVE SOLUTION — To 750 ml saturated aqueous picric acid solution add 250 ml formalin (37%-40%) and 50 ml glacial acetic acid.

CARBOL FUCHSIN SOLUTIONS
    Ziehl Neelsen's — 2.5 ml melted phenol, 5 ml absolute ethyl alcohol, 0.5 gm basic
        fuchsin in 50 ml distilled water.
    Kinyoun's — 4 gm basic fuchsin, 8 ml melted phenol, 20 ml 95% ethyl alcohol, and
        100 ml distilled water.

CARBOL XYLENE CREOSOTE SOLUTION — 10 ml creosote, 10 ml melted phenol in
    80 ml xylene.

CASEIN GLUE — (Ch. 23)

CELLOIDIN SOLUTIONS — (Ch. 13)

CHROMIC ACID (CHROMIUM TRIOXIDE) SOLUTIONS
    4% — 4 gm chromic acid (chromium trioxide) in 100 ml distilled water.
    10% — 10 gm chromic acid (chromium trioxide in 100 ml distilled water.

CITRIC ACID SOLUTIONS
    0.3% — 0.3 gm in 100 ml sterile water.
    1% — 1 gm citric acid in 100 ml distilled water.

COLEMAN'S SCHIFF REAGENT — see Periodic acid-Schiff procedure - (Ch. 18).

COLLOIDAL IRON SOLUTIONS (Muller's)
    Stock — 4.4 ml 29% ferric chloride solution in 250 ml boiling distilled water.
    Working — 20 ml of stock colloidal iron solution, 15 ml distilled water, and 5 ml glacial
        acetic acid.

CONGO RED SOLUTION, 1% — 1 gm Congo red in 100 ml distilled water.

CRESYL ECHT VIOLET SOLUTION, 0.1% — 0.1 gm cresyl echt violet in 100 ml distilled
    water. Add 15 drops of glacial acetic acid just before using. Filter.

CRESYL VIOLET V STOCK SOLUTION — 0.04 gm cresyl violet V, 85 ml distilled water,
    and 15 ml glacial acetic acid.

CRESYL VIOLET V-TRIETHANOLAMINE SOLUTION — Equal parts of cresyl violet V
    solution and 15% triethanolamine solution.

CROCEIN SCARLET - ACID FUCHSIN SOLUTIONS — (Ch. 17)

CRYSTAL (GENTIAN) VIOLET SOLUTIONS
    1% — 1 gm crystal (gentian) violet in 100 ml distilled water.
    Stock, 14% — 14 gm crystal violet in 100 ml 95% ethyl alcohol.
    Working — 10 ml stock 14% crystal violet solution in 300 ml distilled water.

DIASTASE SOLUTION — (Ch. 18)

EOSIN SOLUTIONS

Stock — 1 gm eosin Y, water soluble in 20 ml distilled water, add 80 ml 95% ethyl alcohol.

Working — 1 part stock, add 3 parts 80% ethyl alcohol and 0.5 ml glacial acetic acid for each 100 ml of stain.

EOSIN-PHLOXINE B SOLUTIONS

Stock eosin — 1 gm eosin Y in 100 ml distilled water.

Stock phloxine — 1 gm phloxine B in 100 ml distilled water.

Working eosin-phloxine B solution — 100 ml stock eosin, 10 ml phloxine B solution, 780 ml 95% ethyl alcohol. Add 4 ml glacial acetic acid.

FERRIC AMMONIUM SULFATE SOLUTION, 2.5% — 2.5 gm ferric chloride in 100 ml distilled water. Use mortar and pestle to break up the large crystals of ferric ammonium sulfate.

FERRIC CHLORIDE SOLUTIONS

2% — 2 gm ferric chloride in 100 ml distilled water.

10% — 10 gm ferric chloride in 100 ml distilled water.

29% — 29 gm ferric chloride in 100 ml distilled water.

FEULGEN REAGENT, SCHIFF — (Ch. 18)

FONTANA SILVER NITRATE SOLUTION — (Ch. 20)

FORMALIN SOLUTIONS

1% — 1 ml 37%-40% formaldehyde solution in 99 ml distilled water.

10%, unbuffered — 10 ml 37%-40% formaldehyde solution in 90 ml distilled water.

10%, buffered neutral — 100 ml 37%-40% formaldehyde solution in 900 ml distilled water, add 4 gm sodium phosphate monobasic and 6.5 gm sodium phosphate dibasic (anhydrous).

20% — 20 ml 37%-40% formaldehyde solution in 80 ml distilled water.

FORMALIN, ACETIC ACID — 10 ml of 37-40% formalin, 90 ml distilled water, and 5 ml glacial acetic acid.

FORMALIN, ALCOHOLIC — 10 ml of 37-40% formalin in 90 ml 80% alcohol.

FORMALIN AMMONIUM BROMIDE SOLUTION — 15 ml formalin (37% - 40%), 2 gm ammonium bromide in 85% ml distilled water.

FORMOL CALCIUM SOLUTION — 1 gm anhydrous calcium chloride, 10 ml formalin (37% - 40%), in 90 ml distilled water.

FORMIC ACID SOLUTION — see Sodium citrate formic acid solution.

FOUCHET'S SOLUTION — 25 gm trichloroacetic acid in 100 ml distilled water. Mix thoroughly then add 10 ml 10% ferric chloride.

GALLOCYANIN SOLUTION — 0.15 gm gallocyanin, 5 gm chromium potassium sulfate in 100 ml distilled water.

GELATIN SOLUTIONS, 5%
Adhesive, 5% — 5 gm gelatin dissolved in 100 ml of heated distilled water. Add a pinch of thymol as a preservative.
Warthin Starry, 5% — 5 gm high grade sheet gelatin in 100 ml acidulated water.

GIEMSA SOLUTION — (Ch. 21)

GLUTARALDEHYDE, 8% — (Ch. 24)

GLYCERINE JELLY — (Ch. 19)

GOLD CHLORIDE SOLUTIONS
1% Stock — 1 ml vial in 99 ml distilled water. To break vial of gold chloride first score with a diamond point pencil, then place vial in a large glass-stoppered bottle. Add half of the water (approximately 45 ml), close the cap, and shake vigorously. Once the vial has broken, add the remaining 54 ml of distilled water. Filter.
0.1% — 10 ml of 1% gold chloride stock solution and 90 ml distilled water.
0.2% — 20 ml of 1% gold chloride stock solution and 80 ml distilled water.

HEMATOXYLIN SOLUTIONS
10% Alcoholic — 10 gm hematoxylin in 100 ml absolute alcohol.
Ehrlich's — (Ch. 13)
Harris' — (Ch. 9)
Mayer's — (Ch. 9)
Acid — (Ch. 22)

HYALURONIDASE SOLUTION — (Ch. 18)

HYDROBROMIC ACID SOLUTION, 5% — 5 ml hydrobromic acid in 95 ml distilled water.

HYDROCHLORIC ACID SOLUTIONS
0.1 N — 10 ml 1 N hydrochloric acid solution in 90 ml distilled water.
0.6 N — 50 ml concentrated hydrochloric acid in 950 ml distilled water.
1N — 83.5 ml hydrochloric acid (sp.gr. 1.19) in 916.5 ml distilled water.
5% — 5 ml concentrated hydrochloric acid in 95 ml distilled water.
10% — 10 ml concentrated hydrochloric acid in 90 ml distilled water.

HYDROGEN PEROXIDE SOLUTION, 3% — commercially available.

HYDROQUINONE SOLUTION, 0.15% — 0.15 gm in 100 ml acidulated water.

IODINE SOLUTIONS
Gram's — 1 gm iodine, 2 gm potassium iodide in 300 ml distilled water.
Lugol's — 1 gm iodine, 2 gm potassium iodide in 100 ml distilled water.

IRON HEMATOXYLIN SOLUTIONS, WEIGERT'S
Stock solution A — 1 gm hematoxylin in 100 ml 95% ethyl alcohol.
Stock solution B — 4.0 ml 29% ferric chloride, 95 ml distilled water and 1 ml concentrated hydrochloric acid.

IRON HEMATOXYLIN WORKING SOLUTION, WEIGERT'S — equal parts of Stock solutions A and B, as 100 ml A and 100 ml B. Weigert's iron hematoxylin working solution is reusable for about 2 weeks.

KERNECHTROT SOLUTION — see Nuclear fast red solution.

LIGHT GREEN SOLUTIONS
Stock solution — 0.2 gm light green, SF yellowish in 100 ml distilled water, then add 0.2 ml glacial acetic acid.
Working solution — 10 ml light green stock solution in 50 ml distilled water.

LITHIUM CARBONATE SOLUTIONS
0.5% solution — 0.5 gm lithium carbonate in 100 ml distilled water.
Saturated solution — 1.54 gm lithium carbonate in 100 ml distilled water.

LUXOL FAST BLUE SOLUTION, 0.1% — 0.1 gm luxol fast blue (MBS) in 100 ml of 95% ethyl alcohol. Add 0.5 ml of glacial acetic acid for every 100 ml of stain.

MAY-GRUNWALD STAIN SOLUTION — (Ch. 21)

METANIL YELLOW SOLUTION, 0.25% — 0.25 gm metanil yellow, 100 ml distilled water, and 0.25 ml glacial acetic acid or 1 gm metanil yellow, 400 ml distilled water, and 1 ml glacial acetic acid (optional).

METHENAMINE (HEXAMETHYLENETETRAMINE) SOLUTION, 3% — 3 gm methenamine (hexamethylenetetramine) in 100 ml distilled water.

METHENAMINE SILVER NITRATE SOLUTIONS
Stock solution — To 100 ml of 3% methenamine solution add 5 ml of 5% silver nitrate solution.
Working solution — To 25 ml methenamine silver nitrate stock solution add 25 ml distilled water. Add 4 ml of 5% borax solution.

METHYLENE BLUE SOLUTIONS
Stock solution — 1.4 gm methylene blue in 100 ml 95% ethyl alcohol.
Working solution — 10 ml methylene blue stock solution in 90 ml tap water.

METHYL GREEN PYRONIN SOLUTION — (Ch. 17)

METHYL ORANGE SOLUTION — (Ch. 17)

MICHAELIS VERONAL ACETATE STOCK BUFFER SOLUTION — 9.7 gm sodium acetate, 14.7 gm sodium barbiturate, 500 ml distilled water. Store in refrigerator. (Ch. 22)

MUCICARMINE SOLUTION — (Ch. 18)

NEURAMINIDASE SOLUTION — see Sialidase solution (Ch. 18).

NITRIC ACID SOLUTION, 5% — To 95 ml distilled water add 5 ml nitric acid.

NUCLEAR FAST RED (KERNECHTROT) SOLUTION — 0.1 gm nuclear fast red (Kernechtrot) in 100 ml of 5% ammonium sulfate solution. Heat to boiling, slowly. Cool, filter, and add a grain of thymol as a preservative.

OIL RED O SOLUTION — (Ch. 19)

ORANGE G SOLUTION, 1 % — 1 gm orange G in 100 ml distilled water.

OSMIUM TETROXIDE SOLUTION, 1% — Mix under hood - Highly Toxic. 1 gm osmium tetroxide in 100 ml sodium phosphate working buffer solution. (Ch. 24)

OXALIC ACID SOLUTIONS
    1.5% — 1 .5 gm oxalic acid in 100 ml distilled water.
    2% — 2 gm oxalic acid in 100 ml distilled water.
    5% — 5 gm oxalic acid in 100 ml distilled water.

PARAROSANILINE SOLUTION, 4% — 1 gm pararosaniline hydrochloride, 20 ml distilled water, add 5 ml concentrated hydrochloric acid. (Ch. 22)

PERIODIC ACID SOLUTION, 0.5% — 0.5 gm periodic acid in 100 ml distilled water.

PHOSPHATE BUFFERED SALINE SOLUTION, pH 7.0 - pH 7.6 — 1.48 gm sodium phosphate, dibasic, 0.43 gm sodium phosphate, monobasic, 7.2 gm sodium chloride in 1000 ml distilled water.

PHOSPHATE HYDROCHLORIC ACID SOLUTION — 958 ml distilled water, 42 ml concentrated hydrochloric acid, 13.8 gm sodium phosphate, monobasic.

PHOSPHOMOLYBDIC ACID SOLUTIONS
    5% — 5 gm phosphomolybdic acid in 100 ml distilled water.
    10% — 10 gm phosphomolybdic acid in 100 ml distilled water.

PHOSPHOTUNGSTIC ACID HEMATOXYLIN SOLUTION — (Ch. 14)

PHOSPHOTUNGSTIC ACID SOLUTION, 5% — 5 gm phosphotungstic acid in 100 ml distilled water.

PHOSPHOTUNGSTIC / PHOSPHOMOLYBDIC ACID SOLUTION — 5 gm phosphotungstic acid, 5 gm phosphomolybdic acid in 200 ml distilled water.

PICRIC ACID/ACETONE SOLUTION — 1 gm picric acid in 100 ml acetone.

PICRIC ACID, SATURATED SOLUTIONS
  Aqueous — 2 gm picric acid in 100 ml distilled water.
  Alcoholic — 1 gm picric acid in 100 ml 95% ethyl alcohol.

POTASSIUM DICHROMATE SOLUTION, 2.5% — 2.5 gm potassium dichromate in 100 ml distilled water.

POTASSIUM FERRICYANIDE SOLUTION, 5% — 5 gm potassium ferricyanide in 100 ml distilled water.

POTASSIUM FERROCYANIDE SOLUTIONS
  5% — 5 gm potassium ferrocyanide in 100 ml distilled water.
  10% — 10 gm potassium ferrocyanide in 100 ml distilled water.

POTASSIUM FERROCYANIDE HYDROCHLORIC ACID SOLUTIONS
  Mallory's Iron — equal parts of 5% potassium ferrocyanide solution and 5% hydrochloric acid solution.
  Microincineration — equal parts of 5% potassium ferrocyanide solution and 0.6N hydrochloric acid solution.

POTASSIUM METABISULFITE SOLUTION, 2% — 2 gm potassium metabisulfite in 100 ml distilled water.

POTASSIUM PERMANGANATE SOLUTIONS
  0.15% — 0.15 gm potassium permanganate in 100 ml distilled water.
  0.25% — 0.25 gm potassium permanganate in 100 ml distilled water or 1 gm potassium permanganate in 400 ml distilled water.
  0.3% — 0.3 gm potassium permanganate in 100 ml distilled water or 3 gm in 1000 ml distilled water.
  0.5% — 0.5 gm potassium permanganate in 100 ml distilled water or 5 gm in 1000 ml distilled water.

PROPYLENE GLYCOL SOLUTION, 85% — 85 ml propylene glycol and 15 ml distilled water.

PROTARGOL SOLUTION — (Ch. 14)

PYRIDINE SOLUTION, 10% — 10 ml pyridine in 90 ml distilled water.

PYROCATECHOL SOLUTION, 0.15% — 0.15 gm pyrocatechol in 100 ml acidulated water. A substitute for hydroquinone in the Warthin-Starry procedure for micro-organisms.

SCHIFF FEULGEN REAGENT — (Ch. 18)

SIALIDASE SOLUTION — (Ch. 18)

SILVER NITRATE SOLUTIONS
  0.5% — 0.5 gm silver nitrate in 100 ml distilled water.
  1% — 1 gm silver nitrate in 100 ml distilled water.

5% — 5 gm silver nitrate in 100 ml distilled water.
10% — 10 gm silver nitrate in 100 ml distilled water.
10.2% — 10.2 gm silver nitrate in 100 ml distilled water
20% — 20 gm silver nitrate in 100 ml distilled water.

SIRIUS RED SOLUTION ,1 % — 1 gm sirius red in 100 ml distilled water. Add 0.5 gm
   sodium chloride. Do not filter.

SODIUM BICARBONATE SOLUTION, 5% — 5 gm sodium bicarbonate in 100 ml distilled
   water.

SODIUM BISULFITE SOLUTIONS
   1% — 1 gm sodium bisulfite in 100 ml distilled water.
   4% — 4 gm sodium bisulfite in 100 ml distilled water.

SODIUM CARBONATE SOLUTION, 5% — 5 gm sodium carbonate in 100 ml distilled
   water.

SODIUM CITRATE FORMIC ACID SOLUTIONS
   Stock solution - A — 50 gm sodium citrate in 250 ml distilled water.
   Stock solution - B —125 ml 90% formic acid in 125 ml distilled water.
   Working solution — equal parts of stock solutions A and B.

SODIUM HYDROXIDE SOLUTIONS
   1% — 1 gm sodium hydroxide in 100 ml of 50% ethyl alcohol.
   10% — 10 gm sodium hydroxide in 100 ml distilled water. Add the sodium
   hydroxide slowly because heat is generated that can cause serious burns.

SODIUM IODATE SOLUTION, 1% — 1 gm sodium iodate in 100 ml distilled water.

SODIUM NITRITE SOLUTION, 4% — 4 gm sodium nitrite in 100 ml distilled water.

SODIUM THIOSULFATE (HYPO) SOLUTION, 5% — 5 gm sodium thiosulfate (Hypo) in
   100 ml distilled water.

SORENSON'S BUFFER SOLUTION — (Ch. 24)

SULFURIC ACID SOLUTIONS
   0.3% — To 99.7 ml of distilled water add 0.3 ml sulfuric acid.
   0.5% — To 99.5 ml of distilled water add 0.5 ml sulfuric acid.
   1% — To 99 ml of distilled water add 1 ml sulfuric acid.

TRIETHANOLAMINE SOLUTION, 15% — 15 ml triethanolamine in 85 ml distilled water.

TRIS BUFFER — See Table 22 - 2

TRYPSIN SOLUTION — 0.1 gm trypsin in 100 ml phosphate buffered saline, pH 7.0 —
   pH 7.6.

URANIUM (URANYL) NITRATE SOLUTION, 1% — 1 gm uranium (uranyl) nitrate in 100 ml distilled water.

VAN GIESON SOLUTION — 5 ml of 1% acid fuchsin solution into 95 ml saturated picric acid solution.

VICTORIA BLUE SOLUTION — (Ch. 21)

XYLENE-PEANUT OIL SOLUTION — 1 part peanut oil to 3 parts xylene as 10 ml peanut oil and 30 ml xylene.

ZIEHL NEELSEN'S CARBOL FUCHSIN SOLUTION — see Carbol fuchsin solutions.

CLEANING OF GLASSWARE FOR SILVER TECHNIQUES

Jack B. Wenger

Acid cleaning of glassware is important in argyrophil techniques, e.g., Churukian Schenk, or where specimens are left in a labile silver solution for any length of time, e.g., Fontana-Masson.

Concentrated nitric acid or the commercial chromate-sulfuric acid mixture is recommended for acid cleaning. Exposure to the solution for about 30 seconds should be followed by thorough washing in tap water and rinsing in several changes of distilled water. Use of large quantities of the chromate-sulfuric acid mixture should be avoided. Hydrochloric acid is not recommended, as any residual chloride will precipitate as silver chloride.

Acid cleaning is unnecessary in Grocott's methenamine-silver technique (GMS). The slides in this procedure are exposed to 4% chromic acid for one hour, which provides effective cleaning. In the GMS procedure, however, the entire interior of the staining dish should be exposed to the 4% chromic acid solution.

The use of disposable plasticware is an alternative to acid cleaning. Plastic slide mailers can be used when impregnating slides. Plasticware is especially desirable for mixing solutions in the Warthin-Starry procedures.

CHAPTER 4

FIXATION

Edna B. Prophet

Fixation not only preserves tissues by stopping autolytic changes but allows tissues to remain unchanged by subsequent treatment. Ideally, the tissues are hardened slightly but are not brittle leaving tissue structures in as lifelike a state as possible with minimal shrinkage. Fixation may be accomplished by immersion or perfusion. Fixation should be performed immediately since delay permits autolysis and drying. Freezing prior to fixation can cause major morphological changes. Placing tissue specimens in saline prior to fixation permits autolysis to proceed.

The choice of a fixative is made with several factors in mind, e.g., structures and entities to be demonstrated and the effects of short-term and long-term storage. There are numerous types of fixatives, each with its advantages and disadvantages. Some fixatives are restrictive; others are multipurpose.

Ten percent buffered neutral formalin is considered the best general fixative for pathological specimens because it preserves the widest range of structures, requires a relatively short fixation time, can be used for long-term storage, and penetrates rapidly and evenly without overhardening. Wet tissue specimens can remain in 10% buffered neutral formalin for many months without adverse effects or unwanted precipitates, and it preserves nuclear and cytoplasmic detail adequately. Furthermore, formalin-fixed specimens can be postfixed with another fixative and thus can be used in electron microscopy. Many immunocytochemical reactions can be carried out on formalin-fixed tissues. For these reasons 10% buffered neutral formalin is almost universally used and the Armed Forces Institute of Pathology recommends this fixative to its contributors.

For special studies, a wide variety of fixatives is available. The user should be aware of the advantages and disadvantages of each fixative and the artifacts associated with them. The length of time in the fixative, the size of the specimens to be fixed, and the storage potential are important considerations.

FIXATIVE INGREDIENTS

A. LIQUIDS. The most commonly used liquids, which are used singly or in combination with other liquids or solids, are alcohol, acetone, formalin, glutaraldehyde, and acetic acid. Trichloroacetic acid is used less frequently. In past years trichloroacetic acid served as both a fixative and a decalcifying agent.

ABSOLUTE ALCOHOL preserves glycogen; however, it causes distortion to nuclear detail and shrinks cytoplasm.

COLD ACETONE is preferred when performing certain histochemical studies for enzymes, especially lipases and phosphatases. Acetone is not used as a routine fixative because it causes distortion to nuclei, shrinks cytoplasm, and does not preserve glycogen.

FORMALIN does not precipitate proteins and only slightly precipitates other constituents of the cell. It does not harden or render albumin insoluble and prevents subsequent hardening by alcohols. Formalin neither preserves nor destroys fat. It is a good fixative for complex lipids but has no effect on neutral fats. Although formalin is not the fixative of choice for carbohydrates, it preserves proteins so that they hold glycogen, which is then not easily dissolved. Formalin is ideal for frozen sections.

Formaldehyde is a colorless liquid or gas with a pungent odor. It is an immediate irritant to the eyes, nose, and throat. The skin and respiratory system are particularly affected. Safety precautions include proper ventilation and exhaust, limited or restricted exposure periods, and thorough washing if spilled on the skin.

Although formalin fixation is universally accepted as an ideal fixative, its effect is considered to be a "soft" fixation. Tissue specimens fixed in formalin may show some nuclear "bubbling." Postfixation with acetic acid formalin (AAF) can prevent this effect. This can be easily carried out in automatic tissue processors. The effect produced by AAF is similar to that of heavy metal fixatives. The histologic quality of specimens can be improved by running them back to the aqueous phase, postfixing them in AAF, and then reprocessing. When nuclear "bubbling" is observed, postfixation with AAF will produce brighter hematoxylin and eosin stains, Giemsa stains, and many other special stains. Postfixation provides better preservation of antigens in immunohistologic preparations.

Formalin should not be used with chromates because it readily oxidizes to formic acid. Even though neutralization can be accomplished with calcium carbonate, specimens removed from formalin neutralized in this manner do not retain their pH. Furthermore, calcium carbonate can itself deposit in tissues, leaving areas of "pseudocalcification." To maintain a stable pH for many months and to store specimens for long periods, we recommend formalin that is neutralized with phosphate buffers, e.g., sodium phosphate monobasic and sodium phosphate dibasic.

Formalin used without neutralization or buffers oxidizes to formic acid, which in turn produces acid *formalin hematin pigment* . This pigment can be seen in sites containing blood.

GLUTARALDEHYDE penetrates more slowly than formaldehyde and is useful in electron microscopy and in enzyme histochemistry. There are many variations in the preparation of this fixative, including the percentage of glutaraldehyde, other additives, and buffers. Small blocks of tissues, 1–2 mm in size, fix well at cold temperatures, 1°–4°C, and fixed tissue specimens can be stored in buffer solution for many months. The slow penetration, cold temperature, and the need for a storage medium prevent the use of this fixative in routine diagnostic histotechnology. Electron microscopists, however, are able to use it with continued success.

TRICHLOROACETIC ACID is not used today. It reportedly preserves sulfur containing amino acids, cystine, cysteine, and methionine in protein. This liquid was also used as a decalcifying agent.

ACETIC ACID is never used alone but is often combined with other fixatives that cause shrinkage. Acetic acid penetrates thoroughly and rapidly but lyses red blood cells.

B. SOLIDS. There are a number of solids that are combined with other solids and liquids to improve fixation.

MERCURIC CHLORIDE (corrosive sublimate, bichloride of mercury) penetrates rapidly and precipitates all proteins. It can improve the histologic appearance of tissues. It has two main disadvantages, however—(1) the mercuric crystals, which are deposited in the tissue, must be removed prior to staining and (2) because it is a highly poisonous substance, regulatory practices prohibit its disposal into sewage systems. Zenker's, Helly's, Ridley's, and B-5 contain mercuric chloride.

The technique for disposing of a fixative that contains mercuric chloride depends on precipitation of the mercuric chloride by thioacetamide.

13% THIOACETAMIDE SOLUTION

Thioacetamide .... 13.0 gm
Distilled water .... 100.0 ml

Mix thoroughly and store in a tightly capped bottle. This solution is stable for approximately one year.

ABSTRACTION PROCEDURE

1. To each liter of Zenker's solution add 20 ml of 13% thioacetamide solution. (Our laboratories have not tested this reaction on other fixatives that contain mercuric chloride.)
2. Mix thoroughly.
3. Place under a hood and leave undisturbed for 24 hours or until a precipitate of mercuric sulfide is formed. BE SURE THAT THE CONTAINER IS CAPPED TIGHTLY.
4. Filter the solution through fluted filter paper or a Buchner filter. USE HOOD.
5. The clear filtrate can now be discarded into the sink. The remaining residue that contains the mercuric salt can be stored indefinitely or turned over to a safety official.

POTASSIUM DICHROMATE fixes cytoplasm without precipitation. This ingredient is never used alone. Following fixation, specimens should be washed thoroughly to remove an oxide that forms that cannot be removed later in processing.

CHROMIC ACID (chromium trioxide) is a strong oxidizer that is used with other ingredients. Chromic acid has no effect on fats and penetrates slowly. Using this ingredient leaves tissues in a state where shrinkage may occur at subsequent steps in processing.

OSMIUM TETROXIDE is a very good fixative for small (2-3 mm³) specimens. It preserves fine structures in cells and is therefore used in electron microscopy as a rapid fixative. Vapors of this fixative will preserve blood and tissue films. Osmic acid mixtures are not used in routine diagnostic histotechnology because these mixtures penetrate slowly and unevenly. Furthermore, tissues often crumble if embedded in paraffin. Osmium tetroxide causes interference with many staining methods.

PICRIC ACID when used in combination with other ingredients leaves tissues soft, penetrates well, and precipitates all proteins. Its use necessitates thorough washing because this ingredient will continue to react with the tissue structures and will cause a loss of basophilia.

To summarize, although certain fixatives have special uses, phosphate buffered neutral formalin is the most versatile and practical fixative and is recommended for routine as well as many specialized procedures.

10% BUFFERED NEUTRAL FORMALIN SOLUTION

Formaldehyde, 37% – 40% .... 100.0 ml
Distilled water .... 900.0 ml
Sodium phosphate, monobasic .... 4.0 gm
Sodium phosphate, dibasic (anhydrous) .... 6.5 gm

Store in properly labeled container. Label as HAZARDOUS chemical. The specimen should be completely submerged in 5-10 times its volume of fixative.

REFERENCES

Lillie RD, Fullmer HM. *Histopathologic Technic and Practical Histochemistry.* New York, NY: McGraw-Hill; 1976:31.

Thompson SM, Luna LG. *An Atlas of Artifacts.* Springfield, Ill: Charles C Thomas; 1978:58-60.

❖ CHAPTER 5

TISSUE PROCESSING: DEHYDRATION, CLEARING, AND INFILTRATION

Edna B. Prophet

The three stages of tissue processing—dehydration, clearing, and infiltration—are sequential steps designed to remove the extractable water from tissue specimens and replace it with a medium that solidifies to allow sectioning.

Alcohols—isopropyl or ethyl—are the usual choice for dehydration. Isopropyl alcohol is cheaper than ethyl alcohol and is not on the list of controlled substances . Routine use of graded alcohols from a lower to a higher concentration is standard. Automatic tissue processors enhance the processing of tissue specimens by using heat, vacuum, pressure,and agitation. Processors also allow the three stages to be carried out overnight and without the presence of personnel.

Xylene, one of many clearing agents, is generally used for routine paraffin embedding because of its compatibility with many types and sizes of tissue specimens.

This chapter is concerned with paraffin processing. For eye, bone, and neurological specimens; plastic processing; celloidin; and electron microscopy, see the appropriate chapters. For routine paraffin infiltration, our laboratories use several of the commercially available paraffins. The sequential steps given in the three processing schedules that follow are for small biopsies, routine specimens, and large blocks.

SHORT SCHEDULE (biopsies and small fragments of tissue)

TOTAL PROCESSING TIME - 3 to 4 hours

Minimum fixation time, 3 hours.
1. Rinse very briefly in running water.
2. Hold, if necessary, in 80% alcohol.
3. 95% alcohol, 3 changes, 15 to 20 min. each.
4. Absolute alcohol, 3 changes, 15 min. each.
5. Equal parts absolute alcohol and xylene, 15 min.
6. Xylene, 2 changes, 15 min. each.
7. Paraffin, 3 changes, 15 min. each.
8. Paraffin, under vacuum, 15 to 20 min.
9. Embed.

OVERNIGHT SCHEDULE (for routine specimens using an automatic tissue processor)

TOTAL PROCESSING TIME -14 to 16 hours

1. 80% alcohol, 1 hour.
2. 95% alcohol, 3 changes, 1 hour each.
3. Absolute alcohol, 3 changes, 1 hour each.
4. Xylene, 3 changes, 1 hour each.
5. Paraffin, 3 changes, 1 hour each.
6. Paraffin, under vacuum, 1 hour.
7. Embed.

HAND PROCESSING SCHEDULE (for specimens larger than standard cassette)

TOTAL PROCESSING TIME - 24 hours

Use a large beaker and a rotating head or magnetic stirrer for dehydration and clearing, then transfer to a tissue processor. The following procedure is used by the Neuropathology Laboratory and is designed for hand processing.
Note: Start processing at midmorning.

1. 80% alcohol, 1 hour.
2. 95% alcohol, 3 changes, 2 hours each.
3. Absolute alcohol, overnight.
4. Absolute alcohol, 2 changes, 1 hour each.
5. Xylene, 3 changes, 1 hour each.
6. Paraffin, 2 changes, 2 hours each.
7. Solidify in paraffin.
8. Melt down in the morning.
9. Paraffin, under vacuum, 2 hours.
10. Embed.

To preserve the quality of the first alcohols, the tissues should remain in 60% or 70% alcohol until ready for processing. If this is practiced routinely, the first alcohols (80% and 95%) remain clearer and the percentage of the alcohols more constant.

There are no advantages in taking shortcuts in processing. The results can be poorly and incompletely dehydrated, cleared, and infiltrated specimens, which will cause further problems when sectioning, staining, and examining the tissues.

Automatic processors can malfunction. Problems arising from this include dried specimens, burned specimens, and specimens that have remained in the clearing agent too long . We have found that "dried out" tissues are best improved by reprocessing in the formol-glycol procedure that follows.

METHOD FOR REPROCESSING TISSUE

FORMOL-SODIUM ACETATE (STOCK)

Formaldehyde, 38%-40% .... 10.0 ml
Sodium acetate .... 2.0 gm
Tap water .... 90.0 ml

FORMOL-GLYCEROL WORKING SOLUTION

Formalin-sodium acetate, Stock .... 90.0 ml
Glycerin (glycerol) .... 10.0 ml

PROCEDURE[a]:

1. Place block or specimen in molten paraffin for 1 hour.
2. Xylene, 3 changes, 1 hour each.
3. Absolute alcohol, 2 changes, 1 hour each.
4. 95% alcohol, 2 changes, 1 hour each.
5. Running tap water for 30 minutes.
6. Place in formol-glycerol solution until tissues become soft and pliable with gentle pressure. Tissues may remain in formol-glycerol for up to 8 hours without adverse effect.
7. Reprocess on tissue processor in usual manner.

[a]Tissues from burned patients show no improvement with the formol-glycerol reprocessing. The above procedure may be initiated at any of the steps, e.g., for tissues that remained too long in clearing agent start at step 3.

REFERENCE

Luna LG, ed. Methods for reprocessing dried tissue specimens. *Histo-Logic.*1978;8(2):1 .

CHAPTER 6

SPECIMEN ORIENTATION

Bob Mills

The quality and suitability of a tissue section depend on every step in processing, and each step is quality dependent on the step preceding it. Even with adequate fixation, flawless processing, and expert microtomy, a tissue section can be destroyed by improper embedding, placement, and orientation. The histopathology technician must scrutinize each and every tissue fragment, analyze its structure, and decide how to position the tissue in the block. A comprehensive working knowledge of gross tissue structure and anatomy is a critical requirement of the technician, and explicit communication with the pathologist is a must. A marking system should be used to identify tissues that require special placement. Paper tags can be placed in the cassette or instructions can be written on a cassette surface. Tissue surfaces or margins can be marked with India ink or notched to indicate proper placement. Having the specimen log book available during embedding is a helpful source of information on the type of tissue being embedded.

GENERAL CONSIDERATIONS

Tissue sections are embedded perfectly flat to assure that a complete section will be obtained. Use just enough pressure to hold the section flat against the mold surface. Care must be taken to prevent causing artifacts by rough handling of the specimen.

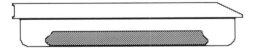 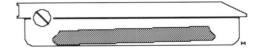

Fig. 6-1

Orientation should be such that the resistance the tissue offers the knife proceeds from the lesser amount toward the greater amount as the block is sectioned. This prevents the harder tissues from compressing the softer tissues above and produces much smoother sections. There must be an adequate margin (2 mm minimum) of embedding medium surrounding all sides of the tissue for maximum cutting support.

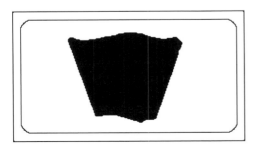 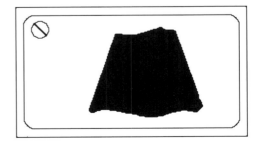

Fig. 6-2

TUBULAR STRUCTURES

Tubular structures such as vas deferens, veins, arteries, and fallopian tubes must be embedded so that the knife cuts across the lumen. Placement should be as vertical as possible. The knife should cut perpendicular to the long axis of the tube.

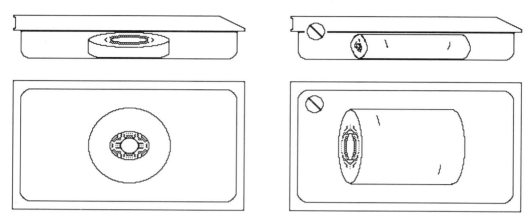

Fig. 6-3

EPITHELIAL SURFACES

Tissues with an epithelial surface such as skin, intestine, gallbladder, urinary bladder, and uterus must be positioned so that the plane of section is across all tissue layers. The epithelial surface should be at the top of the block so that it will be cut last. In most cases, cutting the epithelium at the end of the cutting stroke will minimize pressure distortion of the epithelial layer. Cutting the hard keratin layer of skin last minimizes compression, scratches, and cuts in the subcutaneous layers.

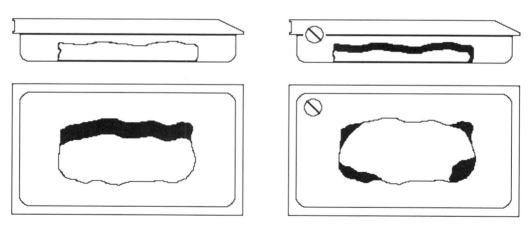

Fig. 6-4

Multiple specimens should be embedded side by side with the epithelial surfaces facing the same direction.

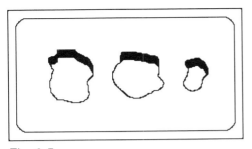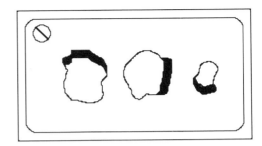

Fig. 6-5

It can be difficult to identify the epithelial surface on very small biopsy specimens. We add 5 ml of stock alcoholic eosin to the second (of 3) 100% alcohol solution on our tissue processor to stain the tissue layers and make the epithelial surfaces easier to visualize. The eosin is washed out of the tissue sections during the rehydration phase and does not interfere with subsequent staining.

LARGE, DENSE SPECIMENS

Large rectangular or dense specimens like uterus, prostate, thyroid, and bone should be embedded at a slight angle to the knife edge. The knife starts the cut with less resistance, reducing the risk of pulling the tissue out of the block. Vibration of the knife edge or block is also notably diminished.

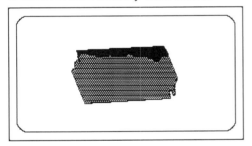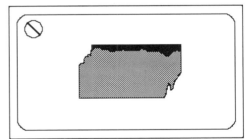

Fig. 6-6

MULTIPLE SPECIMENS

Multiple soft tissue fragments and lymph nodes should be placed side by side with space between them. If tissues are placed one above the other, there is the chance that the lower tissue will distort the upper one. The orderly organization of the tissue makes the slide easier to read and looks much more professional than randomly embedded fragments.

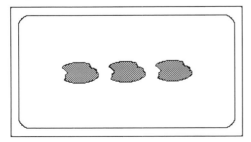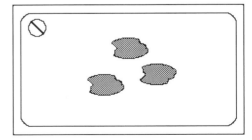

Fig. 6-7

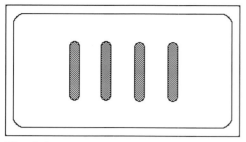 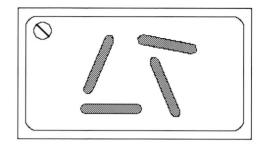

Fig. 6-8

Small rectangular tissues should be oriented with their long axis nearly parallel to the knife edge to minimize pressure distortion and wrinkling.

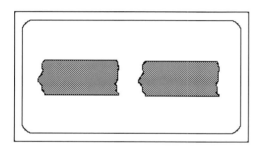 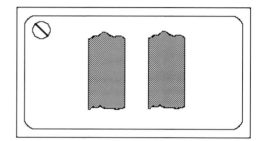

Fig. 6-9

CYSTIC STRUCTURES

Small bisected cysts have a dome shape. The cyst should be embedded with the cut surface down so that the knife cuts through all layers of the cyst wall. Be sure that the dome does not trap air bubbles.

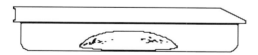 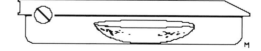

Fig. 6-10

INKED SURFACES AND MARGINS

Tissues that have had the *margins* identified with India ink or dye should be placed so that the ink will be visible on the section (on the edge). Multiple sections should be embedded with the ink facing the same side of the block to make the slide more organized and easier to study.

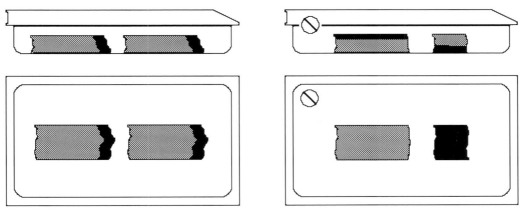

Fig. 6-11

If a *surface* has been marked with India ink, the inked surface should be embedded up, opposite the surface that will be cut by the knife. The ink will not be visible on the sections.

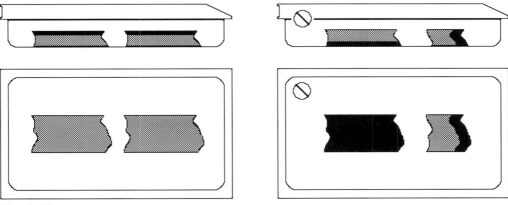

Fig. 6-12

These are only guidelines. The great diversity of tissue types, shapes, and sizes demands constant attention and decision making by an experienced technician.

❖ CHAPTER 7

EMBEDDING

Joe Hall

Embedding is the process of surrounding tissue with a firm substance such as wax to facilitate the cutting of thin sections. While paraffin is the most popular and widely used embedding medium, there are others such as celloidin, ester wax, and water-soluble embedding media.

PARAFFIN EMBEDDING MEDIA

Paraffin is a mixture of solid hydrocarbons derived from petroleum. It is colorless or white, somewhat translucent, odorless, and available with varying melting points. Soft paraffins have a melting point of about 45°C and work best with soft tissues such as fetal or areolar connective tissues. Hard paraffins have a melting point of about 60°C and are optimal for hard tissues such as dense fibrous tissue or bone. Since it is usually impractical for a routine pathology laboratory to separate specimens for embedding in hard or soft paraffin, a paraffin with a melting point of about 56°C is recommended for general purposes. Climate should be considered when choosing paraffins. Soft paraffins are not recommended for use in hot climates because of their low melting point. Stored paraffin blocks made from a soft paraffin are likely to melt if the room temperature exceeds 40°C and should therefore be stored in a cool, dry area.

Plastic polymers are added to paraffin in order to increase consistency and to give it greater elasticity. It causes the paraffin to form ribbons more easily and aids in preventing compression of the sections.

Dimethyl sulfoxide (DMSO) is a hygroscopic, colorless liquid. It is added to promote rapid paraffin infiltration. It is especially useful if vacuum is not available during infiltration.

Rubber is added to paraffin to increase its elasticity and is particularly good for circular specimens because it allows the original shape of the specimen to be regained after sectioning.

Beeswax is mixed with paraffin, in a 10% to 20% proportion of beeswax, in order to give a uniform cutting consistency and the elasticity necessary to obtain wrinkle-free sections.

EMBEDDING EQUIPMENT

There are several specialized materials and equipment that facilitate paraffin embedding.

Embedding molds are used for casting/shaping liquid paraffin into blocks. There are many types. Stainless steel molds are perhaps the most widely used and are considered ideal for embedding purposes. They are manufactured in various sizes to accommodate different sizes of tissue specimens. They are reusable but periodic cleaning is required.

Plastic molds are disposable and therefore, the need for cleaning after use is eliminated. They are very shallow and require an embedding cassette or ring in conjunction with each mold in order to give the block support during sectioning.

Pop-out embedding molds are made of hard aluminum alloy and consist of two sections that are hinged together to form a complete unit. "Legs" are designed to automatically hold the mold in the closed position when in use. For removal of the block, the mold is swung open and the block pops out.

L pieces consist of two L-shaped pieces of metal resting on a flat metal base. The L pieces can be moved to adjust the size of the mold so that it will match the size of the tissue.

Multiblock embedding units allow numerous blocks to be embedded using only one apparatus. It consists of a series of interlocking plates on a tray. The plates create separate compartments, each of which may be used as a mold. By leaving one or more of the plates out, larger blocks may be cast.

Embedding centers are multifunctional units usually equipped with a paraffin dispenser, specimen holding tank, warm plate for orienting the specimen in melted paraffin and a cold plate for transforming the melted paraffin into a solid block after the specimen has been oriented. These can be purchased as one streamlined, modular unit.

PARAFFIN EMBEDDING TECHNIQUE

Using forceps warmed with a commercial forceps warmer or a Bunsen burner to prevent the paraffin from collecting on them, remove a processing cassette that contains the impregnated tissue from the paraffin holding area. Open the processing cassette in order to view the tissue sample. A mold that best corresponds to the size of the tissue sample is selected and partially filled with paraffin. Rewarm the forceps, remove the tissue from the cassette and place it at the bottom of the mold. If the processing cassette is also used as an embedding cassette, the lid should be discarded and the bottom retained for embedding purposes. If the processing cassette is used only to process the specimen, then the entire cassette may be discarded after processing is complete.

Transfer the mold from the warm plate to the cold plate and the wax will quickly form a thin solid layer on the bottom of the mold. Gently press the surface of the tissue to be sectioned against the solid layer which will hold it in the desired position. If multiple pieces are to be embedded, this process must be carried out rapidly, otherwise the paraffin will solidify before each piece of tissue can be properly orientated. (See Chapter 6, Specimen Orientation.)

If an embedding ring or cassette is used, it should be placed firmly on top of the embedding mold at this point. Fill the combined mold and embedding cassette with paraffin and cool immediately by placing the mold on the cold plate of the embedding console. The paraffin should solidify in about 15 minutes; the mold is then separated from the embedding cassette. The tissue and solidified wax remain attached to the embedding cassette, forming a paraffin block that is now ready for sectioning.

If pop-out molds or similar types of molds are used, embedding cassettes or rings are not required. The mold should be filled with paraffin and placed on the cold plate in order for the paraffin to solidify. After approximately 30 minutes (when the paraffin solidifies), the mold should be separated from the paraffin, producing a paraffin block that is now ready for sectioning.

CELLOIDIN EMBEDDING TECHNIQUES

Celloidin is a purified form of nitrocellulose obtained by treating cellulose with sulfuric and nitric acids. It is supplied as a pulpy, cottonlike material and has also been referred to as gun cotton.

In the past it was advantageous to use celloidin rather than paraffin as an embedding medium because it provided better support for hard tissue specimens such as uterus or bone as well as for fragile specimens such as eyes and neurologic tissues. With the introduction of newer types of paraffin, it is no longer advantageous to use celloidin solely for the purpose of good support. Celloidin does not require heat at any stage of processing and therefore is recommended for infiltrating and embedding specimens that would be damaged by heated solutions. This is the one advantage that celloidin still has over paraffin.

Disadvantages of Celloidin
1. The procedure is time consuming, requiring 7 to 10 days to infiltrate a specimen.
2. Celloidin attracts moisture very quickly, which prevents the solution from solidifying and causes the blocks to become too soft to section.
3. The blocks require storing in 70% to 80% alcohol.
4. The knife and block must be kept moist with 70% to 80% alcohol.
5. It is extremely difficult to obtain sections thinner than 10 um.
6. Ether is required, which is extremely flammable.

Advantages of Celloidin
1. It causes less shrinkage and hardening of tissues than does paraffin because there is no heat involved in the process.
2. The relationship of tissue components is well preserved.
3. It is excellent for the study of embryos and large specimens.

Preparation and Use of Celloidin
Celloidin may be supplied in a moistened condition in absolute ethanol or as dry strips; the latter form is preferable but more expensive. If accurate dilutions are to be made, it is recommended that the moistened form of celloidin be dried overnight on filter paper in an incubator at 37°C before it is used. The dried celloidin is then weighed and soaked in absolute ethanol to dissolve it. This is done by dissolving 24 gm of celloidin in 100 ml of absolute ethanol. This solution should be stirred frequently to insure that it is completely dissolved. After the celloidin is dissolved, 100 ml of ether is added to make a 12% solution. Other dilutions of celloidin may be prepared from the 12% solution by using the following chart.

Percentage desired	Parts 12% celloidin	Equal parts of Abs Alc & Ether
10	5	1
8	4	2
6	3	3
4	2	4
2	1	5

Celloidin solutions should be made in advance and kept on hand. They should be stored in glass jars with ground glass stoppers to avoid evaporation of the solvents and contamination with water. One should also be aware of the safety hazards involved when using ether since it is extremely flammable.

Infiltration
Tissue specimens selected for processing with celloidin should be no more than 5 mm in thickness. After the tissue has been properly fixed and dehydrated, the following schedule is used for infiltration with celloidin:

Preparation of Wet Celloidin
1.   Ethyl ether-alcohol, 100%, equal parts ....24 hours
2.   Celloidin, 4% ....2 to 3 days
3.   Celloidin, 8% ....2 to 3 days
4.   Celloidin, 12% ....2 to 3 days
5.   Embed.

Preparation of Dry Celloidin
The dry celloidin technique is used to avoid the necessity of having to cut celloidin blocks using 80% alcohol. The following procedure is used to prepare dry celloidin blocks.
1.   Follow steps 1 through 4 of the wet celloidin method above.
2.   Place tissue in equal parts of cedarwood oil and chloroform for 24 hours
3.   Place in solution of cedarwood oil 3 parts and chloroform 1 part for 24 hours.
4.   Store blocks in cedarwood oil for 24 hours or longer.

Celloidin Embedding Technique
1.   Place the oriented tissue in embedding molds that contain thick 12% celloidin. The molds should measure at least 2 to 3 cm in depth to avoid exposure of the tissue as the celloidin evaporates and shrinks.
2.   The molds are then placed under a sealed bell jar or in a desiccator until all of the air bubbles have disappeared from the celloidin, approximately 12 hours. This procedure may be accelerated if vacuum is applied simultaneously.
3.   After the air bubbles have disappeared, the solution is then hardened by lifting one side of the bell jar or by opening the door to the desiccator, thus exposing the solution to the outside air causing the solvents to evaporate. Hardening of the celloidin may be accelerated by placing a chloroform-soaked cottonball in the bell jar or desiccator, separate from the specimen. The blocks are completely hardened when they are firm to the touch and the finger no longer leaves imprints on the surfaces of the blocks.
4.   For wet celloidin cutting, remove the blocks from the chloroform vapor and place them upside down in 80% ethanol until they are ready to be mounted.

Mounting Blocks for Sectioning
One reason for using celloidin as an embedding medium is to facilitate the sectioning of large specimens; therefore, the blocks may vary in size according to the size of the specimen. It is thus necessary to mount them onto vulcanite or wooden blocks before they can be sectioned on a microtome. The following procedure is used for mounting celloidin blocks:
1.   Trim the celloidin blocks into squares with parallel sides.
2.   Coat the surface of the mounting block with a 2% celloidin solution and firmly press it against the back of the celloidin block. The surface of the mounting block should be roughened to assure adequate adhesion of the celloidin block.
3.   At this point, pressure is applied in the form of a weight or a vise to hold the surfaces of the celloidin and mounting blocks in close contact.
4.   Harden the block in 80% ethanol for about an hour before sectioning.

Low Viscosity Nitrocellulose (LVN)

LVN may be used instead of celloidin for similar purposes. The average impregnation time for LVN is 6 to 11 days. The final LVN block is harder than a celloidin block because LVN is not as viscous. This makes it possible to use higher concentrations. One drawback to using LVN is that the sections have been known to crack during staining. This problem can be avoided if 95% alcohol is used as a solvent instead of absolute alcohol. It is also suggested that a small amount of celloidin be added to the LVN solution (about 1%) to overcome this problem.

WATER-SOLUBLE EMBEDDING MEDIA

Water-soluble embedding media make it possible to take the specimen from the fixative and place it directly into the infiltrating solution. This eliminates the need to dehydrate and clear tissue specimens. Water-soluble media are invaluable when it is necessary to demonstrate entities that would be dissolved by solutions such as xylene or that are rendered inactive by heat. There are various water-soluble embedding media available, including carbowax, gelatin, agar, and Optimum Compound Temperature (O.C.T.) . O.C.T. is the only water soluble-embedding medium routinely used at the AFIP. See Chapter 12, Frozen Sections.

❖ CHAPTER 8

MICROTOMY

Virginia A. Achstetter

This chapter addresses knife sharpening and sectioning. Tissue orientation is covered in Chapter 6.

MICROTOME KNIVES

The selection of a microtome knife (stainless steel, carbide, diamond, glass, or disposable blades) depends on the structure of the specimen to be sectioned and the medium used for embedding.

Stainless steel and tungsten carbide knives are used for sectioning paraffin and resin-embedded specimens, respectively. The lengths of the knives range from 110 mm to 250 mm. The profiles of knives are designed for specific applications. Because of their versatility, our laboratories use profile C knives for routine sectioning.

Fig. 8-1 **Diagram of Profiles**

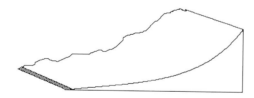

A. Very concave - used for
fresh specimens and soft celloidin.

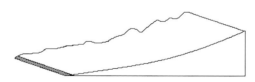

B. Slightly concave - used for soft
paraffin embedded specimens and
harder celloidin.

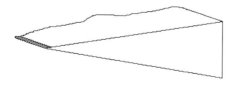

C. Wedge-shaped - used for most paraffin
embedded specimens, hard celloidin, some
plastics.

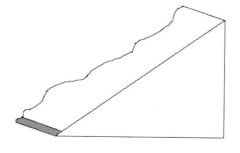

D. Wedge-shaped with steep cutting
edge - used for plastics.

Disposable blades also provide an excellent cutting edge for paraffin sectioning. These are available in different sizes and thicknesses. The stainless steel holder for the disposable blade must be kept clean and well lubricated so that the blade is held securely.

Specimens embedded in resins such as epoxy and glycolmethacrylate require the use of diamond, sapphire, or glass knives that have harder edges. Diamond and sapphire knives are better than glass knives but are more expensive. Glass knives are more often used in electron microscopy laboratories and require skill to make, which may prove to be very tedious and time consuming, especially for the novice.

KNIFE SHARPENING

A well-sharpened knife is free of nicks and "wire edges" and has facets of the same size on either side of the blade. A change in the knife's facet could alter the clearance angle, which may require readjustment of the angle setting. An angle of 5 to 10 degrees is generally optimal (Fig. 8-2). It is important to remember that knives perform best when they are sharpened on the same sharpener each time. Any changes in pressure on the knife against the sharpening surface will affect the cutting edge.

There are many commercial sharpeners available. Sharpeners with a glass plate remove nicks with a coarse abrasive and sharpen and polish with a fine abrasive. Other sharpeners recondition as well as sharpen knives. A disadvantage to reconditioning is that the cutting surface is ground away with each treatment, shortening the life of the knife.

Knife lines account for many of the laboratory generated artifacts seen in slides. Even though care has been taken to insure proper fixation, processing, and embedding a nicked, dull knife can ruin tissue sections.

Fig. 8-2 **Knife bevel and relationship to knife sharpening and cutting**

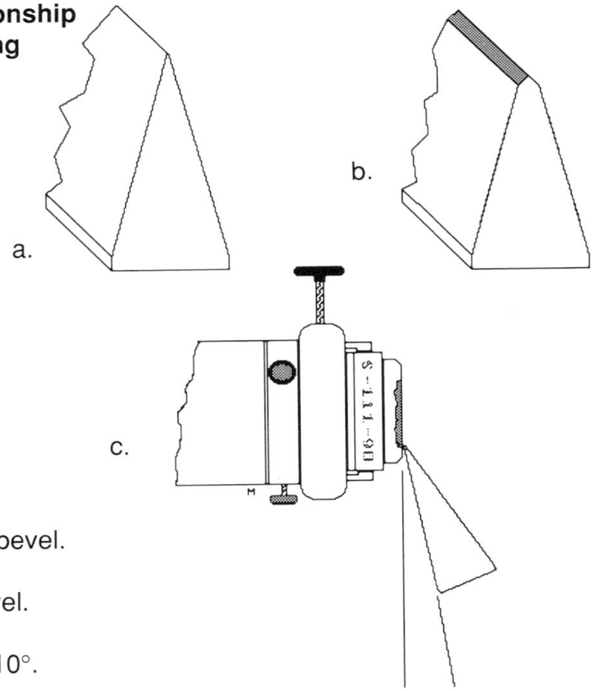

a. Steel knife, side view, without bevel.

b. Steel knife, side view, with bevel.

c. Microtome - angle between 5-10°.

MICROTOMY

Two types of microtomes are used to make thin sections for light microscopy: (1) the rotary microtome, where the block moves, is the most widely used; and (2) the sliding microtome, where the knife moves, is particularly useful when sectioning large blocks, including whole mount preparations.

Section Thickness

For routine tissue sectioning, it is conventional to set the thickness selector at 6 micrometers. In sectioning highly cellular tissues, e.g., lymph nodes, 4 micrometers is appropriate. This reduces overlapping of nuclei. There are certain structures that are best examined in thicker sections, e.g., amyloid at 10 micrometers and myelin at 15 micrometers. Neurological specimens have the widest range of thickness, 6 to 20 micrometers. Elongated tissue elements such as myelinated nerves are best demonstrated by sectioning at 15 to 20 micrometers.

Block Orientation

Correct positioning of properly embedded blocks in the microtome will result in final preparations of the entire surface which are free of tears, lines, folds, or cellular distortion.

Rough Cutting, Soaking, and Chilling

Before sectioning a block, examine it and establish how it should be oriented into the block holder. Trim away the excess paraffin from the sides, leaving greater margins at the top and the bottom of the block. Once the block is secured in the holder, adjust it to insure that it clears the knife. Rough cutting can now begin. If the block is not parallel to the knife, readjust the block holder screws. To rough cut, the block is thick sectioned by repeatedly advancing the block manually and taking a slice, stopping when the entire surface of the tissue is exposed. Place a piece of wet cotton over the surface of the block for 30 seconds to 1 minute. Use water that is at room temperature to lukewarm. Retract the block holder slightly because "soaking" causes the tissue to swell. Next, chill the knife and the block briefly using an ice cube. There are instances when only the knife, not the block should be chilled, e.g., when sectioning brain, spinal cord, and lymph nodes. When brittle or hemorrhagic specimens are encountered, soak the block surface with an alkaline solution such as 10% diluted ammonium hydroxide. This will soften the tissue, prevent cracking, and facilitate sectioning. Calcified tissues may require a brief soak with 10% formic acid solution to facilitate sectioning. (See Chapter 15 for illustrations.)

Ribboning

When creating a ribbon, the handwheel should be turned at a slow and even speed. Rotating the handwheel too rapidly can cause sections of unequal thickness. Place the ribbon onto the surface of the flotation bath as described below.

Flotation

The flotation bath should be heated to a few degrees below the melting point of the paraffin. The use of distilled water in the water bath will help eliminate air bubbles. Tap water may be used (see below). The ribbon is gradually lowered onto the flotation bath to eliminate wrinkles and entrapped air. Air bubbles may be removed with a camel's hair brush or by submerging a slide under the ribbon. The slide is drawn gently under the section containing bubbles and the bubbles are removed. Allow the sections to remain on the water bath until they are flattened. The sections are separated and placed onto clean premarked slides. The slides are drained vertically for several minutes before placing them onto a warming table that is set at 37°C to 40°C where they are to remain overnight. Failure to drain slides will create air bubbles under the tissue and decrease the section's adhesion to the slide. Air bubbles produce section unevenness and staining artifacts making the final preparation difficult to examine with the microscope. When it is not feasible to dry the slides overnight, they should be positioned flat on a metal tray and placed in an oven set at 58°C for 20 to 30 minutes. Allow the slides to cool before staining.

Sealing Blocks

Once the desired sections have been cut, remove the block from the block holder and seal the exposed surface with molten paraffin. This insures that the tissues will not dry out and become hard and brittle and will facilitate resectioning of the blocks weeks, months, and years later.

Section Adhesives

The most common and routinely used section adhesives are gelatin and casein glue. Gelatin is used for routine paraffin work and casein glue for paraffin sections that are followed by immunohistochemical procedures, including those requiring digestion. Gelatin is added to the water bath. Casein glue is applied to clean slides by dipping (see Chapter 23 for method of preparation). The slides are then air dried for later use.

Cleaning

The use of adhesives in the water bath promotes the growth of bacteria and fungi. Daily cleaning of the water bath with sodium hypochlorite solution, e.g., Clorox, soap, and water is necessary to prevent such contamination. A water bath with a removable glass dish that can be cleaned is recommended.

Preparation of Tap Water for Use in Flotation Baths

Tap water used in flotation baths upon which ribbons of tissue sections are floated is prepared as follows:

$$1\% \text{ hydrochloric acid} \dots\dots\dots\dots 20.0 \text{ ml}$$
$$\text{Tap water} \dots\dots\dots\dots 4000.0 \text{ ml}$$

Slowly add acid to water. Bring solution to boiling point. Cool and add to flotation bath as needed.

Boiling the solution removes CO_2 from the tap water which reduces air bubble formation in the flotation bath. The addition of 1% hydrochloric acid prevents the precipitation of mineral salts which occurs after the CO_2 has been boiled off. Precipitated mineral salts deposit as crystals on unstained sections and bind with dyes during the routine and special staining process. This artifact will appear as splotches of dye in stained tissue sections when examined by light microscopy. Also, histologic sections later used for scanning electron microscopy which were floated on water contaminated by precipitated mineral salts render false positive results during mineral detection tests.

Table 8–1

Problems in Sectioning and Possible Causes

1. **Split ribbons or lengthwise scratches**
   Dirt or other undesirable material on knife edge
   Calcium, foreign bodies (sutures or crystals
      in specimens)
   Grit or dirt in paraffin

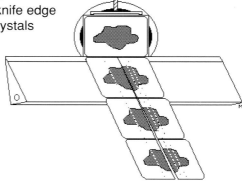

2. **Thick and thin sections**
   Block too large for microtome used
   Loose set screws
   Block or tissue too hard to section
      without soaking
   Tilt of knife insufficient to clear bevel
   Knife holder or disposable blade holder rusted

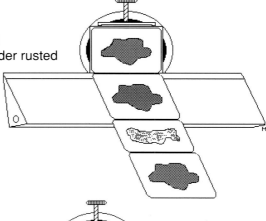

3. **Compressions and wrinkles**
   Knive and/or block warm
   Knife too vertical
   Sections too thin
   Loose microtome set screws
   Dull knife

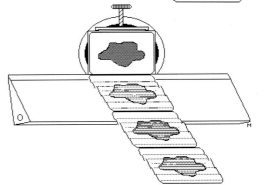

4. **Scratches, lines, or splits in part of section**
     Dirt of foreign bodies in paraffin
     Calcium or foreign bodies in tissue

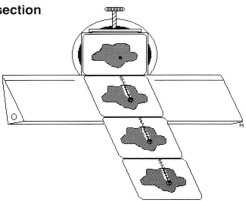

5. **Unequal size sections**
     Block not adequately rough cut or
     aligned with knife.

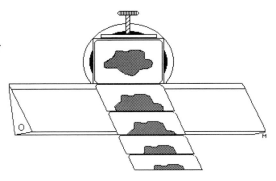

6. **Uneven or crooked ribbons**
     Irregular knife edge
     Knife and block not parallel
     Block not square or rectangular

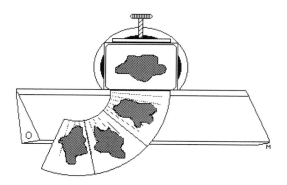

7. **Holes or thick and thin portions in sections**
   Tissue not processed completely

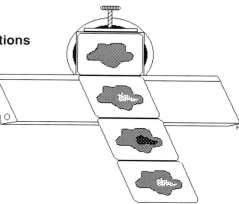

8. **Dry, torn, incomplete sections**
   Incomplete processing or infiltration
   Paraffin too hot at infiltration or embedding stages

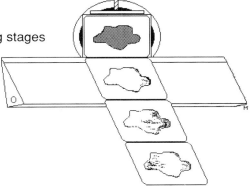

9. **Ribbons will not form**
   Dull knife
   Block too warm
   Incorrect knife angle
   Loose microtome mechanism
   Incomplete tissue processing

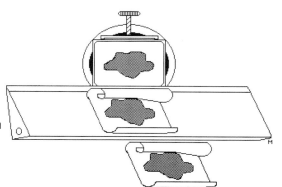

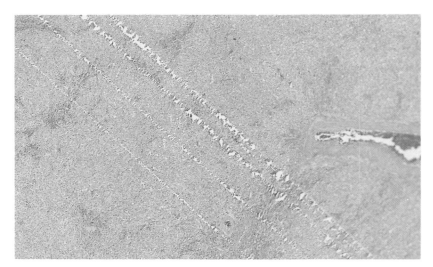

Fig. 8–4. Knife marks resulting from nicks in knife. Gastric lymphoma.

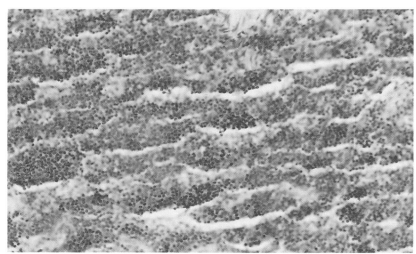

Fig. 8–5. "Venetian blind" (chatter) artifact. This can be caused by erratic rotation of microtome wheel; specimens with both hard and soft components; extremely hard blocks; vibrations in the cutting instrument. Lymph node.

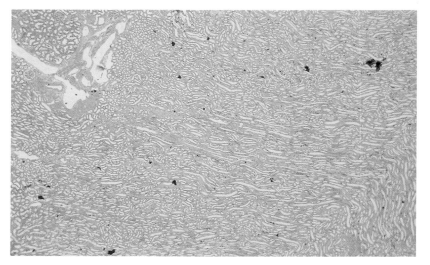

Fig. 8–6. Graphite deposits from soft lead pencils used to mark the slides. Kidney.

❖ CHAPTER 9

HEMATOXYLIN AND EOSIN

Thomas C. Allen

Hematoxylin, a natural dye, was first used around 1863. In combination with aluminum, iron, chromium, copper, or tungsten salts it is an excellent nuclear stain. The active coloring agent, hematein, is formed by oxidation of the hematoxylin. This process, known as "ripening," occurs naturally if hematoxylin solutions are allowed to stand for several days. However, hematoxylin solutions can be used immediately if an oxidizer, sodium iodate or mercuric oxide, is used. Because this oxidation process continues over the life of the hematoxylin solution, solutions should be stored in dark bottles until ready for use. The life of the working solution is variable. Each laboratory at the AFIP uses approximately 800 ml per week. An average of 200 slides can be stained with this volume of solution without noticeable loss of nuclear staining.

Currently, there are two hematoxylin procedures used in the AFIP histopathology laboratories: the Mayer and Harris methods. The Orthopedic Laboratory uses the Harris method, a **regressive** method, since decalcification often reduces the basophilic staining properties in nuclei. This method stains all tissue structures, i.e., nuclei, cytoplasm, connective tissues, etc., and is followed by controlled decolorization and "bluing" to arrive at the optimum nuclear staining results. The other laboratories use Mayer's hematoxylin, a **progressive** procedure that stains the nuclei only. Enhancement of the blue color is accomplished by washing the slides in running tap water. Both of these procedures are described in this chapter. For special notes and critical points in the use of Harris' method, see Chapter 13, Orthopedic Histotechnology.

MAYER'S HEMATOXYLIN STOCK SOLUTION

Ammonium or potassium alum ....50.0 gm
Distilled water..1000.0 ml
Hematoxylin crystals ....1.0 gm
Sodium iodate ....0.2 gm
Citric acid ....1.0 gm
Chloral hydrate ....50.0 gm

Twenty ml of a 2% sodium iodate solution may be substituted for the 0.2 gm of sodium iodate. Add directly to the stock solution after the hematoxylin has dissolved. Dissolve the alum in the distilled water using a magnetic stirrer. When the alum is completely dissolved, add the hematoxylin crystals. When all of the hematoxylin has been dissolved, add the sodium iodate. Let stir for approximately 10 minutes before adding the citric acid. Stir for another 10 minutes before adding the chloral hydrate. Continue stirring until the chloral hydrate is completely dissolved . The resulting solution, if properly prepared, will be a deep "wine" color. One ml of the solution dropped into tepid water will immediately turn blue.

Following the application of hematoxylin, eosin solutions are used conventionally to counterstain. Eosin-phloxine gives the widest range of contrast — pink to bright red. Cytoplasm stains pink and collagen and muscle stain bright red.

EOSIN STOCK SOLUTION

Eosin Y, water soluble .... 1.0 gm
Distilled water .... 100.0 ml

PHLOXINE STOCK SOLUTION

Phloxine B .... 1.0 gm
Distilled water .... 100.0 ml

EOSIN-PHLOXINE WORKING SOLUTION

Combine in a 1000-ml cylinder:
Eosin stock solution .... 100.0 ml
Phloxine stock solution .... 10.0 ml
Alcohol, 95% ethyl .... 780.0 ml
Acetic acid, glacial .... 4.0 ml

The solution is good for approximately 1 week.

Fig. 9-1 Stain line

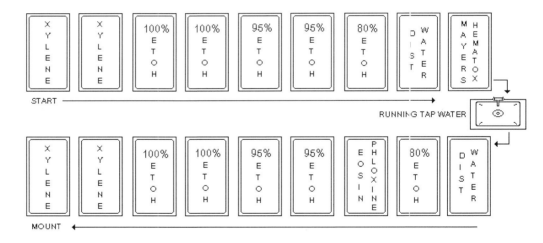

MAYER'S HEMATOXYLIN AND EOSIN PROCEDURE

FIXATION: 10% buffered neutral formalin, Bouin's or Zenker's

SECTIONS: Paraffin, 3 to 8 micrometers.

SOLUTIONS
MAYER'S HEMATOXYLIN (see above)
EOSIN-PHLOXINE SOLUTION (see above)

PROCEDURE (See Fig. 9-1)
1. Deparaffinize slides and hydrate to water. Dezenkerize, if necessary, before staining.[a]
2. Stain in Mayer's hematoxylin solution for 15 minutes.
3. Wash in lukewarm running tap water for 15 minutes.
4. Place in distilled water.
5. Place in 80% ethyl alcohol for 1 to 2 minutes.[b]
6. Counterstain in eosin-phloxine solution for 2 minutes.
7. Dehydrate and clear through 2 changes each of 95% ethyl alcohol, absolute ethyl alcohol, and xylene, 2 minutes each.
8. Mount with resinous medium.

RESULTS
Nuclei ....blue
Cytoplasm ....pink to red
Most other tissue structures ....pink to red

[a]If tissues have been in a fixative containing mercuric chloride, remove pigment before going on to step 2. See below for "dezenkerization" procedure.

[b]The 80% ethyl alcohol at step 5 preserves the strength of the eosin-phloxine solution.

HARRIS' HEMATOXYLIN AND EOSIN PROCEDURE

FIXATION: 10% buffered neutral formalin, Bouin's or Zenker's.

SECTIONS: Paraffin, frozen or celloidin, 3 to 20 micrometers.

SOLUTIONS

1% ACID ALCOHOL (Ch. 3)

AMMONIA WATER (Ch. 3)

SATURATED LITHIUM CARBONATE (Ch. 3)

EOSIN-PHLOXINE SOLUTION (see above)

HARRIS' HEMATOXYLIN

Hematoxylin ....5.0 gm
Alcohol, 100% ethyl ....50.0 ml
Potassium or ammonium, alum ....100.0 gm
Distilled water...1000.0 ml
Mercuric oxide, red ....2.5 gm

Use a 2000-ml flask for the alum and water and a small flask for the alcohol and hematoxylin. Completely dissolve the alum in the distilled water with the aid of heat and a magnetic stirrer. Vigorously shake to dissolve the hematoxylin in the alcohol, at room temperature. Remove the alum and distilled water from the heat. Slowly combine the two solutions. Return the combined solutions to the heat. Bring to a boil as rapidly as possible, approximately 1 minute or less. Remove from the heat and slowly add the mercuric oxide. If the mercuric oxide is added too rapidly, the reaction will cause the solution to boil up and out of the flask. Return the solution to the heat until it becomes a dark purple, remove it from the heat, and plunge it into a basin or sink of cold water to cool. The solution is ready for use. Add 20 ml of glacial acetic acid to intensify the nuclear stain. Always filter before each use.

PROCEDURE

1. Deparaffinize slides and hydrate to distilled water. Dezenkerize, if necessary, before staining.
2. Stain in freshly filtered Harris' hematoxylin for 6 to 15 minutes.
3. Wash in running tap water for 2 to 5 minutes.
4. Differentiate in 1% acid alcohol, 1 to 2 dips.
5. Wash briefly in tap water.
6. Place in weak ammonia water or saturated lithium carbonate solution until sections are bright blue.
7. Wash thoroughly in running tap water for 10 minutes.
8. Place in 80% ethyl alcohol for 1 to 2 minutes.
9. Counterstain in eosin-phloxine solution for 2 minutes.
10. Dehydrate and clear through 2 changes each of 95% ethyl alcohol, absolute ethyl alcohol, and xylene, 2 minutes each.
11. Mount with resinous medium.

RESULTS

Nuclei ....blue
Cytoplasm ....pink to red
Most other tissue structures ....pink to red

REMOVAL OF MERCURY PRECIPITATE PIGMENT
"Dezenkerization"

SOLUTIONS

GRAM'S IODINE SOLUTION (Ch. 3) or

LUGOL'S IODINE SOLUTION (Ch. 3)

5% SODIUM THIOSULFATE (HYPO) SOLUTION (Ch. 3)

PROCEDURE

1. Deparaffinize and hydrate slides to distilled water.
2. Place slides in Gram's or Lugol's iodine solution for 15 minutes.
3. Rinse in tap water.
4. Place in 5% sodium thiosulfate (hypo) solution for 3 minutes.
5. Wash thoroughly in tap water for 10 minutes
6. Stain as desired.

REFERENCE

Sheehan DC, Hrapchak BB. *Theory and Practice of Histotechnology*. Columbus, Ohio: Battelle Press; 1980:153-154.

CHAPTER 10

MOUNTING MEDIA

Thomas C. Allen

The final step in the preparation of a slide is to cover the portion containing the tissue with thin glass, a coverslip. This makes the slide permanent and permits microscopic examination. To affix the coverslip, mounting media of three types can be used: natural resins, synthetic resins, and aqueous media.

Of the natural resins, Canada balsam was the standard in the past; however, its long drying time makes it impractical for routine use. Furthermore, it may reduce the intensity of eosin staining after several years and can cause poor preservation of basic aniline dyes and early fading of Prussian blue reactions. For these reasons, our laboratories use synthetic resins as mounting media for routine hematoxylin and eosin preparations and for most special stains.

Aqueous media (below) are employed when dyes or structures are altered or destroyed by dehydration or by xylene-based media., e.g., lipid stains. Furthermore, dyes such as crystal violet lose their metachromasia in the dehydration and clearing steps.

GLYCERIN JELLY

Gelatin ....10.0 gm
Distilled water...60.0 ml
Heat until the gelatin is dissolved.
Add:
Glycerin ....70.0 ml
Phenol ....1.0 ml

APATHY'S MOUNTING MEDIUM

Acacia (gum arabic) ....50.0 gm
Cane sugar (sucrose) ....50.0 gm
Distilled water...150.0 ml
Sodium chloride ....10.0 gm
Thymol ....0.1 gm

Mix the acacia, cane sugar, and distilled water in a flask. Place the flask in a pan of boiling water until the ingredients are dissolved. Dissolve the sodium chloride and thymol in this solution. Filter with a Seitz filter while the solution is still warm or use a coarse filter paper and place in a 60°C oven, changing filter paper frequently. Refrigerate to remove air bubbles.

POLYVINYL ALCOHOL MOUNTING MEDIUM

The modified polyvinyl medium has been used successfully following procedures for lipid stains on frozen sections and some immunohistochemical procedures; however, it is not recommended for use following amyloid stains and eosin dye procedures. A small quantity of this medium can be kept at room temperature in a dropper bottle for use. The stock solution, however, is stored in the refrigerator. Discard the solution if it becomes lumpy.

          Polyvinyl alcohol (Vinol 205) ....20.0 gm
          Buffered phosphate saline, pH 7.2-7.4 ....80.0 ml
     Heat to 50°C to 60°C and stir for 16 hours using a magnetic stirrer.
     Add:
          Glycerin ....50.0 ml

Stir until the solution is uniform. Add several crystals of thymol as a preservative. Filter the warm mixture through a fritted glass funnel, using coarse filter paper. Wash funnel immediately in hot water. To reduce air bubbles, store upside down in the refrigerator in an airtight container. Warm small quantities to room temperature and dispense as you would any mounting medium. Do not dilute.

COVERSLIPPING: Important Considerations

1. Choose the proper size
   coverslip for specimen.

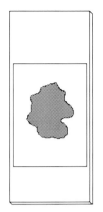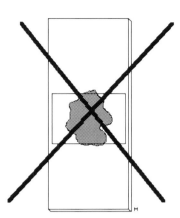

Fig. 10-1

2. "Roll" coverslip onto slide to expel trapped air.

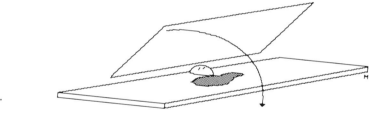

Fig. 10-2.

3. Clean excess mounting medium from edges
   of coverslip with lint-free tissue or gauze
   moistened with the appropriate solvent.
   Avoid smearing the viewing area.

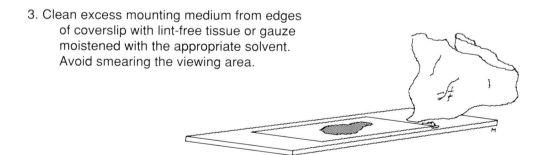

Fig. 10-3.

❖ CHAPTER 11

SLIDE REFURBISHING AND REPAIRS

Gayle G. Andre

This chapter covers the restaining of sections and repair of broken slides. Both require coverglass removal.

COVERGLASS REMOVAL
1. Place slide in xylene until the coverslip slides off. This can be time consuming. For more rapid removal place the slides in xylene in a 56°C to 60°C oven for 15 to 20 minutes. The gradual warming will soften the resinous mounting media, and the coverslips can be easily removed. The method of passing the slides over an open flame is not recommended. Serious burns to the mounted tissue and to the technologist can result.
2. Dissolve the residual mounting medium by gently placing the slides, in staining racks, in several changes of xylene. Do not agitate.

RESTAINING
To restain or refurbish old and faded slides, including those with deteriorated mounting medium, begin with steps 1 and 2, the coverglass removal procedure, and then follow steps 3 through 6 below.
3. Hydrate through several changes of absolute ethyl alcohol, 95% ethyl alcohol to distilled water.
4. Decolorize slides in 1% acid alcohol (see Ch. 3) solution, if necessary.
5. Wash thoroughly to remove the residual acid alcohol.
6. Restain as indicated: H&E to H&E or H&E to special stain.

REPAIR OF SLIDES:
1. If the slide is broken but the coverglass is intact, attach the broken slide to a new blank slide using plastic cement that is not soluble in xylene, e.g. Duco Cement. Allow to dry overnight.

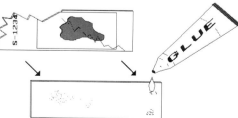

Fig. 11-1

2. Remove the coverglass by soaking in xylene.

3. Rinse in several changes of xylene to remove the residual mounting medium.

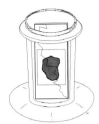

Fig. 11-2 and 3

4. Pour USP flexible collodion over the section and allow the excess to run off from a vertical position.

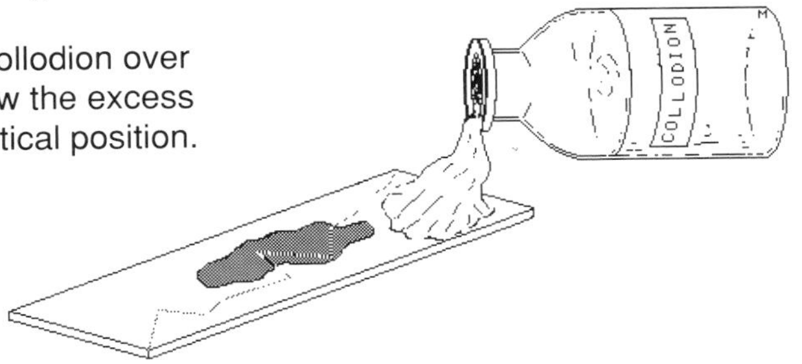

Fig. 11-4

5. Allow the slide to dry thoroughly for several hours or immerse the almost-dry slide briefly in chloroform to hasten the removal of solvent and then dry.

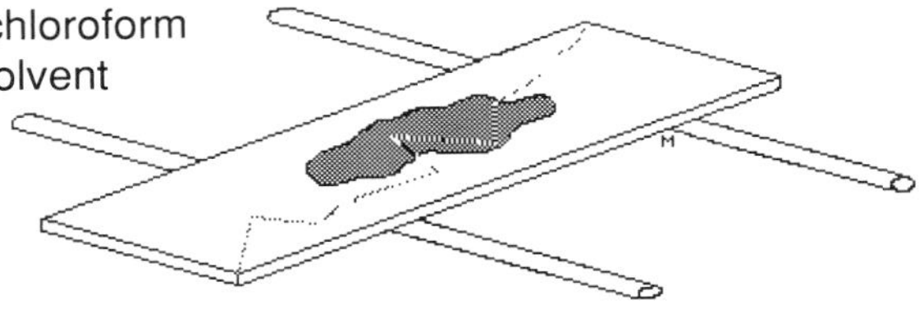

Fig. 11-5

6. Soak the dry slide in distilled water until the collodion coating loosens. This may take 5 minutes to 1 hour.

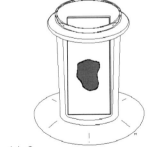

Fig. 11-6

7. Slide a sharp razor blade under an end of the collodion film, then lift off the film and section with fine forceps.

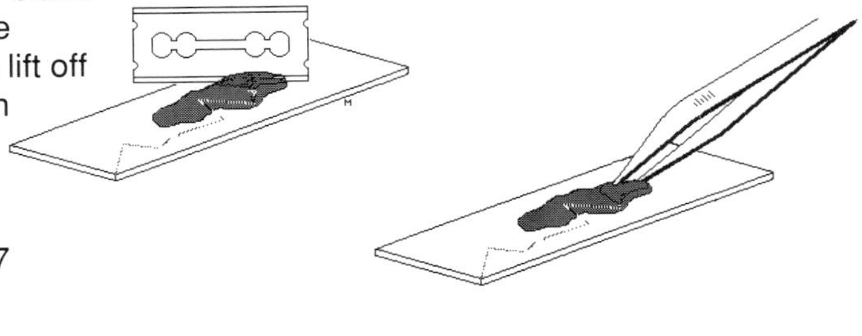

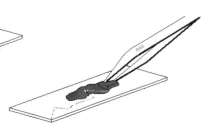

Fig. 11-7

AFIP Laboratory Methods in Histotechnology

8. Place the film and section onto a clean blank slide that has been coated with albumin or another adhesive.

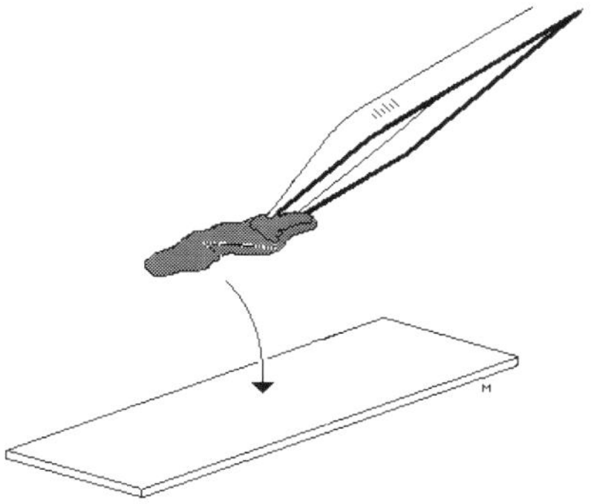

Fig. 11-8

9. Carefully remove the collodion coating with multiple changes of acetone.

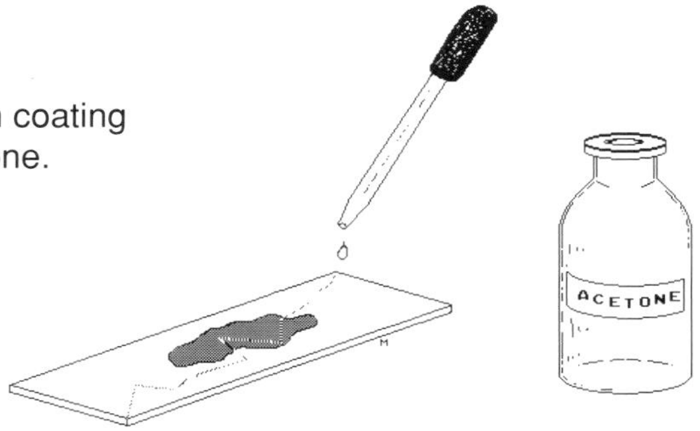

Fig. 11-9

10. Mount using resinous mounting medium.

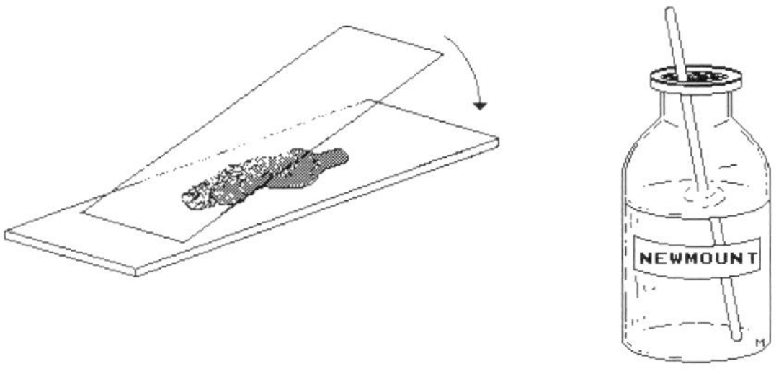

Fig. 11-10

REFERENCE

Johnson FB. Foreign substances in tissues. In: *Histochemistry in Pathologic Diagnosis.* Spicer SS, ed. New York, NY: Marcel Dekker; 1986, p 107.

CHAPTER 12

FROZEN SECTIONS

Bob Mills

For rapid diagnosis or for performing various special stain techniques, fresh or fixed tissues are frozen in lieu of being routinely processed and sectioned. Using carbon dioxide to freeze the tissue, sectioning can be accomplished on a clinical freezing microtome or on the mechanically refrigerated cryostat. Since the clinical freezing microtome method is difficult to master, has numerous disadvantages, and is generally considered outmoded, this chapter will deal only with the use of the cryostat.

THE CRYOSTAT

A cryostat consists of a rotary type microtome enclosed in a mechanically refrigerated cabinet; virtually, it is a microtome in a deep freeze. Many cryostats have platforms or chambers on which to rapidly freeze tissue, and most have self-defrosting capability. In the cryostat's controlled environment, the microtome, microtome knife, cabinet interior, and instruments are all maintained at the same operating temperature so that the sectioning operation is rarely affected by room temperature. The freezing platforms or chambers eliminate the need to use liquid nitrogen or other freezing agents for the vast majority of tissue types. Elimination of liquid nitrogen and agents like dichlorotetrafluoroethane (canned freeze sprays) is an important safety consideration and helps reduce operating costs.

CRYOSTAT MAINTENANCE

The cryostat is a precision instrument and must be properly maintained for optimal performance. All moving parts must be kept clean, adjusted correctly, and lubricated with a low-temperature lubricant as specified by the manufacturer. Operating temperature should be checked, adjusted when necessary, and recorded daily. Ice accumulated on the cabinet interior should be removed daily since it acts like a blanket of insulation, causing the refrigeration unit to work harder. Even the self-defrosting cryostats need manual defrosting occasionally, especially in very humid environments. Ice crystals on the moving parts can make the mechanism stiff and difficult to use. The ice should be removed with absolute alcohol and the moving parts lubricated. Tissue debris should be removed after each case is completed, as tissue fragments can adhere to the mechanism and knife and can contaminate another tissue sample or slide.

CRYOSTAT KNIVES

Section quality is directly related to the condition of the knife edge. In our laboratories we routinely use standard wedge-shaped microtome knives and have had excellent results with some of the new disposable knife systems. For safety reasons, we prefer to use the shorter 125 mm knives and always fit the exposed edges with knife guards. We sharpen our knives on a glass plate style knife sharpener with liquid abrasives and achieve superb results. If a disposable knife system is used, the blade must be cleaned before it is mounted in the knife holder. Most disposable blades are coated with silicone or oil which can be removed with xylene followed by absolute alcohol. Knife angle is important but seems to be a little less critical than in the paraffin technique.

TEMPERATURE

Each type of tissue has an optimum cutting temperature, but it is impossible, especially during sectioning for rapid diagnosis, to adjust the cryostat temperature for every tissue. Our machines are set at -20°C and perform adequately for most tissues. The cabinet, microtome, microtome knife, and any tools (forceps, paintbrushes, etc.) must all be at the same temperature. It is a good idea to keep a spare sharp microtome knife stored in the cabinet so that if your regular knife becomes dull or nicked you can instantly change knives without regard for cool-down time.

SECTION ADHESIVES

Adhesives are infrequently necessary when performing an H&E stain on fresh tissue. The proteins in the tissue and tissue fluids coagulate in the first alcohol or fixative and help the section adhere to the slide. Sections of fixed tissue have a greater tendency to float off of the slide, and many special stain techniques will loosen both fresh and fixed tissues. Thorough washing of fixed tissues before sectioning can also help prevent section loss. If the sections just will not stay put, several adhesives may be used, providing that the adhesive does not interfere with the stain to be performed. Some of the common adhesives for frozen sections are:

MAYER'S EGG ALBUMIN SOLUTION

Egg whites ....50.0 ml
Glycerine ....50.0 ml

Apply a thin layer to the slide just before use.

CHROME ALUM GELATIN SOLUTION

Gelatin, type A, 275 Bloom ....3.0 gm
Chromium potassium sulfate ....0.5 gm
Distilled water ....1000.0 ml

Heat the water to 60°C and completely dissolve the gelatin with the aid of a magnetic stirrer. Stir in the chromium potassium sulfate. (The solution should turn a pale blue.) Add a few crystals of thymol as a preservative. Dip clean slides in the warm solution, blot the edges, and then stand the slides on end to air dry. Once dried, store in dust-free container until ready for use.

10% CASEIN GLUE SOLUTION (Ch. 23)

Some texts mention the use of 0.5% celloidin ether mixture to coat the tissue section before staining. Because of the explosive nature of celloidin and ether, we have discontinued its use.

CUTTING TECHNIQUE

1. A small amount of a liquid embedding medium such as Tissue Tek II O.C.T. is spread evenly on the appropriate object holder. The tissue is placed on the surface of the object holder and completely surrounded with embedding medium. The embedding medium should provide adequate support for sectioning and have at least 2-mm margins (Fig. 12-1). Care must be taken to orient the tissue properly.

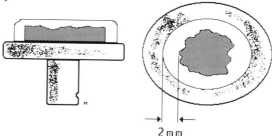

Fig. 12-1   2 mm

2. The object holder is placed on the freezing platform in the cryostat to start the freezing process. If necessary, more embedding medium is added as the tissue freezes. The freezing process can be accelerated if the object holder is at -20°C, the same temperature as the cryostat chamber.

3. When the tissue is completely frozen, the object holder is securely mounted to the microtome head.

4. Preliminary "facing" of the tissue:
   - a. Adjust the knife holder so that the tissue just clears the knife.
   - b. Release the automatic advance pawl from the toothed ratchet wheel.
   - c. Manually advance the ratchet wheel until the tissue extends over the knife edge approximately 0.1 - 0.5 mm. The exact distance will be easy to estimate with experience.
   - d. Release the lock on the drive wheel (large hand wheel).
   - e. Rotate the drive wheel counter clockwise 180° to cut the "rough" tissue section. Immediately return the drive wheel to the upright position.
   - f. Repeat steps c. through e. until the desired cutting plane is reached. Lock the drive wheel.

5. Engage the automatic advance pawl and the toothed ratchet wheel. Carefully clean the knife edge with dry gauze.

6. Unlock the drive wheel. Slowly and smoothly rotate the wheel clockwise. As the section begins to form on the knife edge, a cold paintbrush may be used to gently guide the section down the face of the knife to help keep the section flat (Fig.12-2). Some machines have plastic anti-roll devices attached to guide the section over the knife.

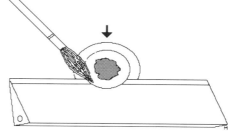

Fig. 12-2

❖ Frozen Sections   69

7. Mount the section on the slide by bringing the surface of a room-temperature slide very close to the section. The section will seem to jump on to the slide, and the mounting medium will melt immediately. There are several suction devices available commercially to assist in holding the slide at the correct angle, but with practice the bare hand is much quicker.
8. The slide is ready to be placed in fixative or to stain.
9. Remember to lock the drive wheel and to clean the tissue debris from the cabinet, mechanism, and knife.

STAINING

The following rapid hematoxylin and eosin procedure is used at the AFIP's Tri-Service School of Histopathology on all surgical specimens that have been sectioned at 6 micrometers.

1. Place fresh tissues in alcoholic formalin for 15 seconds.
2. Dip 10 times in 70% ethyl alcohol.
3. Rinse well in distilled water.
4. Stain in Harris hematoxylin for 45 seconds to 1 minute.
5. Rinse well in tap water.
6. Dip 3 times in saturated lithium carbonate solution or until the section turns blue, approximately 30 seconds. (Weak ammonia water may be substituted for the saturated lithium carbonate solution.)
7. Rinse well in tepid tap water.
8. Counterstain in eosin/phloxine solution for 30 seconds.
9. Begin dehydration with 5 quick dips in each of 2 changes of 95% ethyl alcohol.
10. Complete dehydration and clearing in 2 changes of absolute ethyl alcohol and 2 changes of xylene, 10 dips in each solution.
11. Mount with resinous medium.

CHAPTER 13

ORTHOPEDIC HISTOTECHNOLOGY

John R. Kammerman, Edna B. Prophet, and Carlton F. Barnes

For routine histotechnology of bone, it is necessary to remove the calcium salts without severely altering cellular detail. Paraffin embedding is recommended for specimens of all sizes, including whole-mount preparations of long bones. A discussion of celloidin processing of temporal bone is included at the end of this chapter.

FIXATION

Fix all tissue samples in 10% buffered neutral formalin for up to 5 days. It is recommended that the large long bones also be wrapped in muslin or several layers of gauze to ensure contact between the entire specimen and the fixative and to prevent fragments of tissue from floating free.

After preliminary fixation, large specimens can be cut to fit into the standard sized cassettes. The long bones of the leg and arm are conventionally sectioned or cut using a band saw.

Additional fixation in double-strength formalin is recommended, especially for whole-mount specimens after sawing.

20% BUFFERED NEUTRAL FORMALIN SOLUTION

Formaldehyde, 37%-40% ....20.0 ml
Distilled water ....80.0 ml
Sodium phosphate, monobasic ....4.0 gm
Sodium phosphate, dibasic ....6.5 gm

Specimens from biopsies and curettages are fixed for 1 to 2 hours in the 20% formalin solution; routine surgical specimens, that would normally fit into the plastic cassettes, 24 to 48 hours; and larger whole-mount specimens such as long bones, 72 hours or longer.

All fixed specimens from biopsies and curettages are washed in slowly running tap water for a minimum of 30 minutes. Larger specimens are washed up to a maximum of 1 hour. Avoid rinsing in rapidly running tap water. To avoid losing small biopsy and curettage specimens carefully decant the fixative.

DECALCIFICATION

8% HYDROCHLORIC ACID STOCK SOLUTION

Hydrochloric acid, concentrated ....80.0 ml
Distilled water ....920.0 ml

8% FORMIC ACID STOCK SOLUTION

       Formic acid ....80.0 ml
       Distilled water ....920.0 ml

HYDROCHLORIC ACID/FORMIC ACID WORKING SOLUTION
Combine equal parts of the 8% hydrochloric acid solution and the 8% formic acid solution.

Procedure
1. Specimens should be decalcified in hydrochloric acid-formic acid working solution 20 times their volume.
2. Change to fresh solution each day until decalcification is complete.
3. Wash specimens thoroughly up to 1 hour.

Specimens should not be crowded together in order to provide for complete decalcification. Overdecalcification can permanently damage a specimen. The following procedures help determine the correct end-point of decalcification.

End-Point of Decalcification
The end-point of decalcification can be checked by specimen x-ray examination, chemical testing, or physical testing. X-ray is the most accurate way to determine when decalcification is complete. If it is not possible to x-ray the specimen, the following chemical test for the presence of residual calcium is recommended over the less accurate and potentially damaging physical tests.

Chemical Test
The following solutions are needed to chemically test for residual calcium.

5% AMMONIUM HYDROXIDE STOCK

       Ammonium hydroxide, 28% ....5.0 ml
       Distilled water ....95.0 ml

5% AMMONIUM OXALATE STOCK

       Ammonium oxalate ....5.0 gm
       Distilled water ....95.0 ml

AMMONIUM HYDROXIDE/AMMONIUM OXALATE WORKING SOLUTION
Use equal parts of the 5% ammonium hydroxide solution and the 5% ammonium oxalate solution.

Procedure
1. Insert a pipette into the decalcifying solution containing the specimen.
2. Withdraw approximately 5 ml of the hydrochloric acid/formic acid decalcification solution from under the specimen and place it in a test tube.
3. Add approximately 10 ml of the ammonium hydroxide/ammonium oxalate working solution, mix well and let stand overnight.

4. Decalcification is complete when no precipitate is observed on two consecutive days of testing. Repeat this test every two or three days.

Physical Tests

The physical tests include bending the specimen or inserting a pin, razor, or scalpel directly into the tissue. The disadvantage of inserting a pin, razor, or scalpel is the introduction of tears and pinhole artifacts. Slightly bending the specimen is safer and less disruptive but will not conclusively determine if all calcium salts have been removed. After checking for rigidity, wash thoroughly prior to processing.

PROCESSING

All specimens are processed using a closed system processor with vacuum such as the Vacuum Infiltration Processor (VIP). The alternating pressure vacuum option is ON for all stations. The schedules that follow correspond to biopsy, surgical, and large specimens.

Table 13-1

PROCESSING SCHEDULES USED IN THE ORTHOPEDIC LABORATORY

	24 HOUR (Biopsy)	48 HOUR (Surgical)	72 HOUR (Large)	TEMP
70% Isopropyl alcohol	1 hr	2 hrs	4 hrs	37°C
80% Isopropyl alcohol	1 hr	2 hrs	4 hrs	
95% Isopropyl alcohol	2 hrs	3 hrs	5 hrs	
95% Isopropyl alcohol	2 hrs	3 hrs	5 hrs	
95% Isopropyl alcohol	2 hrs	3 hrs	5 hrs	
100% Isopropyl alcohol	2 hrs	5 hrs	7 hrs	
100% Isopropyl alcohol	2 hrs	5 hrs	7 hrs	
100% Isopropyl alcohol	2 hrs	5 hrs	7 hrs	
Xylene	2 hrs	5 hrs	7 hrs	
Xylene	2 hrs	5 hrs	7 hrs	
Paraffin, 56°C	3 hrs	5 hrs	7 hrs	60°C
Paraffin, 56°C	3 hrs	5 hrs	7 hrs	60°C
Vacuum				

Ethyl alcohol can be used in processing, but it is a controlled substance.

EMBEDDING

Paraffins that contain plastic polymers such as Ameraffin, 55°C to 57°C, are preferred. The plastic polymers cause the paraffins to have a degree of hardness that approximates that of bone. The multiple-pan embedding method is preferred. There are very few occasions when plastic cassettes are used, with the exception of small biopsy specimens.

SECTIONING
Depending on the size of the specimen, there are several choices of microtomes in routine use: the standard rotary for biopsy and surgical specimen blocks, and the sliding for larger and whole-mount specimens. Special types of microtomes are available to section small undecalcified plastic-embedded specimens of bone. When selecting a microtome, consider its resistance to vibration.

H&E STAINING

SOLUTIONS

HARRIS' HEMATOXYLIN (Ch. 9)

1% ACID ALCOHOL SOLUTION (Ch. 3)

SATURATED LITHIUM CARBONATE SOLUTION (Ch. 3)

EOSIN-PHLOXINE SOLUTION (Ch. 9)

PROCEDURE
For bone specimens only
1. Deparaffinize and hydrate to distilled water, 2 changes each of xylene, absolute ethyl alcohol, and 95% ethyl alcohol, 3 minutes each.
2. Stain in freshly filtered Harris' hematoxylin for 10 minutes.
3. Wash in running tap water for 5 minutes.
4. Dip quickly once in 1% acid alcohol solution.
5. Wash in running tap water for 5 minutes.
6. Blue sections in saturated lithium carbonate solution for approximately 5 seconds.
7. Wash in running tap water for 4 minutes.[a]
8. Counterstain in eosin-phloxine solution for 2 minutes.
9. Dehydrate and clear through 2 changes of 95% ethyl alcohol, absolute ethyl alcohol, and xylene, 2 minutes each.
10. Mount with resinous medium.

RESULTS
Nuclei .... blue
Cytoplasm and other tissue structures .... pink to red

[a] Marble chips or limestone can be added to the containers of running water to reduce the acidity of the water, since, in some cases, tap water will decolorize the nuclear stain.

TEMPORAL BONE HISTOTECHNOLOGY

Temporal bone specimens, which include bone anterior to the internal auditory meatus and extend posteriorly into the mastoid region, contain the delicate structures of the middle and inner ear. The procedures outlined below are recommended for use in order to preserve these delicate structures and to minimize technical artifacts including shrinkage and distortion. To remove the specimen block from the skull, which contains both the middle and inner ear structures, a first cut is made perpendicular to the tentorial attachment anterior to the internal auditory meatus. A second cut is made perpendicular to the tentorial attachment, one and one-half inches posterolateral to the first cut. These cuts, if extended three-fourths of an inch anterolaterally and inferiorly, will contain all of the middle ear and inner ear bone anterior to the internal auditory meatus and posterior into the mastoid region.

FIXATION
1. Place specimen in 20% buffered neutral formalin for 24 hours, changing the solution several times during the first hour. Insure that trapped air is removed by gentle agitation. If it is necessary to handle or maneuver the specimen, use forceps. A volume 400 ml to 500 ml of fixative is adequate for a pair of temporal bones.
2. Transfer specimen to 10% buffered neutral formalin for 24 hours.
3. Place in a fresh change of 10% buffered neutral formalin.
4. If trimming is needed, use a circular or band saw. Then place the specimen in a tall specimen jar and agitate vigorously in 10% buffered neutral formalin to remove sawdust and tissue debris.
5. Tissues may be held at this point in tightly capped specimen jars or processed through decalcifying solution.

Solution

1% NITRIC ACID IN 10% FORMALIN SOLUTION

Nitric acid, concentrated .... 1.0 ml
Formalin solution, 10%, unbuffered .... 99.0 ml

To prepare 1000 ml of solution add 10 ml of concentrated nitric acid to 990 ml of 10% formalin solution.

Procedure
1. Suspend the specimens in decalcification fluid measuring 20 times their volume. Never allow a specimen to rest on the bottom of the container. A specimen can be wrapped and secured in a gauze pouch or suspended by a nylon suture or wax-coated string inserted through a soft tissue area, tied securely, and tagged with an identifying number.
2. Change decalcifying solution each day.
3. After 2 or 3 weeks, test the last change of decal solution for the presence of calcium salts (see Chemical Test for decalcification above).
4. Place specimen in 5% sodium sulfate solution for 24 hours.

5. Wash in water for 48 to 72 hours. Use water that is bubble free to avoid entrapping air. For human temporal bones, 20 to 30 days are required for decalcification.

PROCESSING

Table 13-2

MANUAL PROCESSING SCHEDULE FOR TEMPORAL BONE

80% Ethyl alcohol, 3 changes, 24 hours each
95% Ethyl alcohol, 2 changes, 24 hours each
100% Ethyl alcohol, 2 changes, 24 hours each
100% Ethyl alcohol ethyl ether, 2 changes, 24 hours each[a]
6% Nitrocellulose (celloidin), minimum time, 3 weeks
12% Nitrocellulose (celloidin), minimum time, 3 weeks
20% Nitrocellulose (celloidin), minimum time, 3 weeks
30% Nitrocellulose (celloidin), minimum time, 3 weeks
35% Nitrocellulose (celloidin) until firm[b]

35% Nitrocellulose solution is prepared as follows:
    Nitrocellulose, 30% ....100.0 ml
    Nitrocellulose, dry ....5.8 gm

[a] Processing specimens into celloidin involves the use of highly explosive ingredients. Be sure that all electrical outlets and other fixtures have been grounded. Insure that there are no sparks or open flames from burners, etc . Prepare under hood.

[b] The firmness matches that of firm gelatin.

EMBEDDING
1. Pour 35% nitrocellulose into Stender dishes.
2. Add a few drops of ethyl ether/absolute alcohol (1:1). Ether alcohol is highly flammable. Use with extreme caution
3. Cover tightly and secure with weights; let stand for 4 to 5 hours. Allow bubbles to escape.
4. Add a few more drops of the ether alcohol mixture to remove the surface bubbles.
5. Up to four temporal bones can be embedded in each large Stender dish.
6. Transfer the specimens, with the identifying tags attached, to the Stender dish containing 35% nitrocellulose.
7. Replace the weights and allow to remain for 3 weeks. Remove weights during the day and replace weights at night. If the humidity in the room is very high, 50% or above, do not remove weights for the entire period.

8. Check the embedding medium for even and uniform consistency throughout. Ideally the surface will not be tacky and will yield slightly to touch. If a crust forms on the surface, reseal and replace the weights. The solvent, ether alcohol, will rise and soften the surface.
9. Flood the surface with chloroform and immediately replace the cover and the weights.
10. Allow to harden for 2 or 3 days. Avoid a shift of specimens if more than 1 specimen is in the dish. Mark the outside of the container with an identifying number.
11. Pou' off chloroform and add enough 80% alcohol to fill the dish. Let stand for 1 day.
12. Cut out individual blocks after checking the identifying numbers. If more than 1 specimen is present, notch a V with a thin-bladed scalpel until the specimen blocks are separated.
13. Store in 80% ethyl alcohol until ready to section. Never allow the specimens to dry, even after sectioning the blocks. Unstained sections are stored in 80% alcohol.

MOUNTING: Use fiber or wooden blocks.
1. Prepare the celloidin block by submerging the underside, the side away from the specimen, in 1/8 inch to 1/4 inch of ether alcohol. Moderate softening of the side to be mounted is necessary to securely affix the specimen to the wooden or fiber block.
2. Wrap a piece of paper around the fiber or wooden block so that approximately 1 cm is extending at the top and forms a cuff.
3. Remove cuffed blocks from the container and pour in thick nitrocellulose.
4. Quickly and firmly press the specimen block onto the wooden or fiber block. Hold firmly for approximately 1 minute.
5. Allow to sit for 5 to 10 minutes.
6. Lift the mounted specimen blocks by holding the wooden or fiber portion and place in 80% alcohol for 24 hours to harden.
7. Remove paper and store in 80% alcohol.

SECTIONING
The equipment required includes a sliding microtome, a sharpened 250-mm steel blade, and several containers of 80% ethyl alcohol.
1. Set the micrometer at 24.
2. Section serially, staining every 10th section with Ehrlich's hematoxylin working solution. The groups of nine unstained sections are placed on numbered pieces of white unglazed filter paper such as Batman manifold paper.

H&E STAINING

EHRLICH'S HEMATOXYLIN STOCK SOLUTION

Hematoxylin, crystals ....5.0 gm
Alcohol, absolute, ethyl ....250.0 ml
Distilled water..250.0 ml
Glycerin ....250.0 ml
Acetic acid, glacial ....25.0 ml
Potassium alum ....50.0 gm

Dissolve the crystals of hematoxylin in the absolute ethyl alcohol, then add the glacial acetic acid and the glycerin. In a 2000 ml flask dissolve the potassium alum in the distilled water. When the alum is completely dissolved, add the combined hematoxylin, alcohol, glycerin, and acetic acid mixture. Loosely cover the mouth of the flask using filter paper. Allow to ripen for approximately 3 months. Avoid direct sunlight.

EHRLICH'S HEMATOXYLIN WORKING SOLUTION

Ehrlich's hematoxylin, stock ....20 to 30 drops
Distilled water ....300.0 ml

Use freshly diluted solution on control slides to test staining reaction. Add a few more drops of Ehrlich's stock solution if nuclei are not adequately stained.

AMMONIUM HYDROXIDE SOLUTION

Ammonium hydroxide ....3 drops
Distilled water ....200.0 ml

OR

DILUTE LITHIUM CARBONATE SOLUTION

Lithium carbonate ....2 to 5 gm
Distilled water ....200.0 ml

EOSIN Y SOLUTION STOCK SOLUTION

Eosin Y ....2.0 gm
Alcohol, 95%, ethyl ....50.0 ml

EOSIN Y WORKING SOLUTION

Eosin Y solution, stock ....6.0 ml
Distilled water ....150.0 ml

PINE OIL/ALCOHOL SOLUTION

Alcohol, 95% ethyl alcohol ....50.0 ml
Pine oil ....50.0 ml

PROCEDURE

1. Place sections in Ehrlich's hematoxylin working solution overnight. Discard.
2. Blue in cold tap water or weak ammonium hydroxide solution or weak lithium carbonate solution.
3. Wash thoroughly in distilled water.
4. Counterstain in eosin Y working solution for 5 minutes.
5. Begin dehydration in 2 changes of 95% ethyl alcohol, 5 minutes each.
6. Place sections in equal parts 95% ethyl alcohol and pine oil.
7. Clear in pine oil for 15 minutes.
8. Place section onto slide.
9. Blot dry with lint-free filter paper.
10. Mount #1 coverglass with balsam or synthetic resin.

RESULTS

Nuclei ....blue
Background ....pink to red

AFIP Laboratory Methods in Histotechnology

❖ CHAPTER 14

NEUROPATHOLOGICAL HISTOTECHNOLOGY

Arnicia E. Downing

The basic histological techniques for central nervous system (CNS) specimens are essentially the same as for specimens from other parts of the body. However, there are significant differences in fixation time and embedding and sectioning techniques along with specific special stain procedures designed to demonstrate structures seen only in brain and spinal cord.

To better understand the various elements which are seen in the CNS, a brief discussion of the component structures will assist the technologist in the selection, performance, and quality control of the special stains performed on CNS specimens.

The nerve cell body of a neuron contains a nucleus and a nucleolus, which are demonstrated with a routine hematoxylin and eosin stain. In the cytoplasm of some of the cell bodies are Nissl bodies, which contain ribonucleic acid granules seen as ribosomes on electron microscopy. Nissl bodies can be demonstrated selectively using cresyl violet (Vogt's method) or gallocyanin (Einarson's method) or with aldehyde thionin/PAS. The method of choice at the AFIP is the cresyl violet method. It is possible to demonstrate inclusion bodies in the cytoplasm of some neurons; e.g., Lafora bodies seen in certain types of epilepsy (periodic acid-Schiff method) and Negri bodies as seen in rabies (Bosch's method for Negri bodies). Neurofibrils are cytoplasmic structures in some neurons and can be demonstrated using a modified Bielschowsky procedure. Other structures that are seen in stained preparations following the modified Bielschowsky include senile plaques, nerve fibers, and nerve endings.

Extending from the cell body of the neuron are one or more processes called axons and dendrites. The unipolar neurons have one process as seen in the dorsal root ganglion cell. Bipolar neurons have one axon and one dendrite as in first order olfactory cells. Multipolar neurons by far outnumber the bipolar and unipolar neurons and are characterized by their numerous dendritic processes, as in the ventral gray matter of the spinal cord and in the Purkinje cells in the cortex of the cerebellum. Neurons and their processes are demonstrated by the Bodian, the Holmes, and the modified Bielschowsky methods. Of these three silver procedures, the Bodian method uses a silver protein, Protargol; the Holmes and Bielschowsky methods use silver nitrate solutions.

Surrounding the axon may be found a complex lipid sheath called myelin. To demonstrate myelin, two procedures are recommended, the Klüver-Barrera method for myelin and nerve cells, which uses Luxol fast blue, and Woelke's method which employs iron hematoxylin.

There are other cells in the CNS which are not involved in the receipt, correlation, and transmission of impulses. These include the neuroglia, ependyma, and epithelia. The functions of these structures and cells include nutrition, support, and phagocytosis.

The vascular and ependymal structures are easily demonstrated with hematoxylin and eosin. To distinguish between the three types of glial cells, special staining procedures are required. Astrocytes and oligodendroglia, sometimes called macroglia, are the main forms of neuroglia. Microglia are migratory cells which serve as phagocytes. Astrocytes bring nutrition to the neurons, and oligodendroglia are responsible for the formation of myelin. Astrocytes are most often demonstrated by Russell's phosphotungstic acid hematoxylin procedure (PTAH) and a modified Holzer method for glial fibers. The Cajal method for astrocytes is employed when frozen sections are available. Penfield's method for oligodendroglia and microglia, when performed on frozen sections, will stain both types of cells black.

To fix the brain adequately, we recommend that the whole brain be placed in 20% buffered neutral formalin for 24 hours, then placed in 10% buffered neutral formalin for 7 to 10 days. Alternately, 10% buffered formalin can be used for the entire procedure. The brain is then ready for gross sectioning. To minimize the fumes from the formalin, one may place the whole brain in 80% alcohol just prior to gross examination. The 80% alcohol also starts dehydration. When grossing has been completed, the specimens not selected for processing should be returned to 10% buffered neutral formalin.

The processing schedules differ for newborn/baby brain and adult brain, whole brain, and muscle/nerve biopsies (Table 14 -1).

As with other types of tissue specimens, brain and spinal cord should be embedded as flat as possible. However, excessive pressure should not be used while pressing the neurological tissues flat. Chilling or freezing of the specimens should be avoided since these actions cause cracking artifacts on sectioning. The paraffin should be allowed to cool slowly at room temperature. Completing the solidification of the paraffin should be accomplished by running cold water over it. Bubbles in the paraffin will cause spaces which, in turn, cause lines crossing through the tissue slices. There are several significant differences in the sectioning of neurological specimens compared to other tissues. The paraffin blocks should never be frozen or the surface of the exposed tissue chilled with an ice cube or refrigerant. Only the knife should be cooled. Once the ribbon has been obtained, the sections or ribbons should be placed on a water bath set at 43°C to which gelatin has been added. Ribboning is made easier if the excess paraffin is trimmed away from the sides of the block. The sides should be trimmed very close to the tissue, though cutting into the specimen should be avoided. The technologist should first try to obtain a ribbon without soaking the block. If unsuccessful, the exposed surface of the block should be soaked with cotton dipped in room-temperature tap or distilled water. Oversoaking should be avoided as it causes the tissue to swell excessively. If oversoaked thin slices are mounted onto slides, these sections will inevitably come off during staining.

Many neurological special stain procedures require a specific section thickness: Bodian and Bielschowsky's procedures need 8-micrometer sections; Luxol Fast blue, Woelke's, cresyl violet, Hirsch-Peiffer, and Congo red require 20-micrometer sections. If special stains are requested on nerve specimens only, the suggested thickness is 15 micrometers

A number of the traditional neurohistological techniques have been supplanted in recent years by immunohistological procedures which are more specific markers of cell type, e.g., glial fibrillary acidic protein (GFAP) for astrocytes.

Table 14 -1

PROCESSING SCHEDULES
Neuropathology Laboratory, AFIP

	BABY BRAIN	ADULT BRAIN SPECIMENS	WHOLE MOUNT SLICES	BIOPSIES MUSCLES & NERVES
Alcohol,[a] 70%	24 hr	--	24 hr	30 min
Alcohol, 80%	24 hr	24 hr	24 hr	30 min
Alcohol, 95% 3 changes	2 hr each	2 hr each	8 hr each	15 min each
Absolute alcohol 3 changes	2 hr each	2 hr each	8 hr each	15 min each
Equal parts of absolute alcohol and xylene	2 hr	2 hr	8 hr	15 min
Xylene 2 changes	2 hr each	2 hr each	8 hr each	15 min each
Paraffin[b] 3 changes[c]	2 hr each	3 hr each	8 hr each	15 min each

[a]Use **ethyl alcohol** only in the above schedules.

[b]Paraplast or Federal Stock embedding compound, melting point 56°C to 58°C.

[c]Place specimens in vacuum oven for a minimum of 1 hour if the tissue processor does not have vacuum.

CRESYL VIOLET (VOGT'S) METHOD FOR NISSL SUBSTANCE

FIXATION: 10% buffered neutral formalin.

SECTIONS: Paraffin, 6 to 20 micrometers.

SOLUTIONS

2 % CRESYL ECHT VIOLET STOCK SOLUTION

Cresyl echt violet ....2.0 gm
Distilled water..100.0 ml

SODIUM ACETATE BUFFER SOLUTION

Sodium Acetate ....2.0 gm
Distilled water..1000.0 ml
Acetic acid, glacial ....3.0 ml

CRESYL ECHT VIOLET WORKING SOLUTION

Cresyl echt violet Stock, 2% solution ....1.0 ml
Buffer solution ....100.0 ml

PROCEDURE

1.   Deparaffinize and hydrate to second change of absolute alcohol.
2.   Place in absolute alcohol for 2 hours.
3.   Place in cresyl echt violet working solution for 40 to 60 minutes.
4.   Differentiate rapidly in 95% alcohol.
5.   Dehydrate and clear through absolute alcohol and xylene, 2 changes each, 2 minutes each.
6.   Mount with resinous medium.

RESULTS   (See Fig. 14–1, page 105).

Nissl substance ....intense purple
Nuclei ....purple
Background ....clear

GALLOCYANIN (EINARSON'S) METHOD FOR NISSL SUBSTANCE

FIXATION: 10% buffered neutral formalin, Zenker's or Zenker-formol.

SECTIONS: Paraffin, 6 micrometers.

SOLUTIONS

GALLOCYANIN SOLUTION

Gallocyanin ....0.15 gm
Chromium potassium sulfate (alum) ....5.0 gm
Distilled water ....100.0 ml

Dissolve the chrome alum in warm distilled water. Add the gallocyanin and boil gently for 10 minutes. Cool and filter. Solution keeps well for one week.

PROCEDURE
1. Deparaffinize and hydrate to distilled water.
2. Place in the gallocyanin solution for 1 hour in a 56°C oven or leave overnight at room temperature.
3. Rinse in distilled water.
4. Dehydrate and clear through 95% ethyl alcohol, absolute ethyl alcohol, and xylene, 2 changes each, for 2 minutes each.
5. Mount with resinous medium.

RESULTS   (See Fig. 14–2, page 105).
Nissl substance ....blue

REFERENCE
Einarson L. A method for progressive selective staining of Nissl and nuclear substance in nerve cells. *Am J Pathol.* 1932;8:295.

MODIFIED ALDEHYDE-THIONIN PAS FOR NISSL SUBSTANCE

FIXATION: 10% buffered neutral formalin.

SECTIONS: Paraffin, 6 micrometers.

SOLUTIONS

0.5% SULFURIC ACID WATER SOLUTION (Ch. 3)

0.5% POTASSIUM PERMANGANATE SOLUTION (Ch. 3)

2% POTASSIUM METABISULFITE SOLUTION (Ch. 3)

ALDEHYDE THIONIN SOLUTION

Thionin ....0.5 gm
Alcohol, ethyl, 70% ....91.5 ml
Paraldehyde ....7.5 ml
Hydrochloric acid ....1.0 ml

Ripen in a tightly stoppered container 3 to 5 days before using.

0.5% PERIODIC ACID SOLUTION (Ch. 3)

SCHIFF'S REAGENT (Ch. 18)

1% ORANGE G SOLUTION (Ch. 3)

5% PHOSPHOTUNGSTIC ACID SOLUTION (Ch. 3)

1% ACETIC ACID SOLUTION (Ch. 3)

PROCEDURE
1. Deparaffinize and hydrate to distilled water.
2. Place in equal parts of the 0.5% sulfuric acid water and the 0.5% potassium permanganate solutions for 2 minutes.
3. Bleach in the 2% potassium metabisulfite solution for 1 minute.
4. Wash well with distilled water.
5. Stain in aldehyde thionin solution, in a covered and tightly sealed dish, for a minimum of 50 minutes.
6. Rinse in distilled water.
7. Oxidize in 0.5% periodic acid for 5 minutes.
8. Rinse in distilled water.
9. Place in fresh Schiff's reagent for 15 minutes.
10. Wash well in running tap water for 15 minutes.
11. Stain in 1% orange G solution for 3 minutes.

12. Place in 5% phosphotungstic acid solution for 1 minute.
13. Rinse briefly in 1% acetic acid solution.
14. Dehydrate and clear through 95% ethyl alcohol, absolute ethyl alcohol, and xylene, 2 changes each, for 2 minutes each.
15. Mount with resinous medium.

RESULTS

Nissl substance ....blue

This procedure is a modification of the stain for the cells of the anterior pituitary gland and pancreatic islet cells.

REFERENCE
Paget GE, Eccleston C. Simultaneous specific demonstration of thyrotroph, gonadotroph and acidophil cells in the anterior hypophysis. *Stain Technol.* 1960;35:120.

BIELSCHOWSKY METHOD FOR NEUROFIBRILS
AFIP Modification

FIXATION: 10% buffered neutral formalin.

SECTIONS: Paraffin, 8 micrometers.

SOLUTIONS

20% SILVER NITRATE SOLUTION (Ch. 3)

AMMONIUM HYDROXIDE, CONCENTRATED

1% AMMONIUM HYDROXIDE SOLUTION (Ch. 3)

10% FORMALIN SOLUTION, UNBUFFERED (Ch. 3)

NITRIC ACID, CONCENTRATED

CITRIC ACID

DEVELOPING SOLUTION

Formalin, 10% unbuffered ....20.0 ml
Distilled water ....100.0 ml
Nitric acid, concentrated ....1 drop
Citric acid ....0.5 gm

5% SODIUM THIOSULFATE (HYPO) (Ch. 3)

PROCEDURE
1. Deparaffinize and hydrate to distilled water.
2. Place in prewarmed (37°C) 20% silver nitrate solution.
3. Stain at 37°C for 15 minutes.
4. Pour off 20% silver nitrate solution. Save in a flask.
5. Place slides in distilled water.
6. To the silver nitrate solution in flask, add 6.0 ml of concentrated ammonium hydroxide.
7. Clear the silver, which at this point is black, by adding, drop by drop, 1 to 3 ml of concentrated ammonium hydroxide until the precipitate that forms clears. Do not use more than 10 ml of ammonium hydroxide. Excess ammonia may cause a precipitate or result in a poor impregnation of the fibers.
8. Pour this ammoniacal silver on the slides and stain for 15 minutes in 37°C oven.
9. Place slides in 1% ammonium hydroxide solution for 1 to 3 minutes.
10. Return this ammoniacal silver to a flask. Add 10 to 25 drops of the developing solution. Place slides in this solution for 3 to 5 minutes.

11. Dip slides in 1% ammonium hydroxide solution to stop the silver reaction. Check microscopically.
12. If fibers are not dark enough, dip in 1% ammonium hydroxide solution before returning to ammoniacal silver developing solution for 3 minutes.
13. Rinse in 1% ammonium hydroxide solution for 3 minutes.
14. Pour on 5% sodium thiosulfate solution and allow to remain for 5 minutes.
15. Rinse in 3 changes of distilled water, 5 minutes each.
16. Dehydrate and clear through 95% ethyl alcohol, absolute ethyl alcohol, and xylene, 2 changes each, for 2 minutes each.
17. Mount with resinous medium.

RESULTS   (See Fig. 14–3, page 105).
Neurofibrils and senile plaques ....black
Background ....yellow to brown

REFERENCE
Mallory FB. *Pathological Technique*. New York, NY:Hafner;1961:158-180.

BODIAN'S METHOD FOR NERVE FIBERS AND NERVE ENDINGS

FIXATION: 10% buffered neutral formalin.

SECTIONS: Paraffin, 8 micrometers.

SOLUTIONS

1% PROTARGOL (PROTEINATE ARGENATE)[a] SOLUTION

Protargol ....1.0 gm
Distilled water ....100.0 ml

Using an acid-cleaned dish, prepare as follows: Sprinkle the Protargol on the surface of the water. Let stand until all the Protargol dissolves. Add 6 gm Copper Shot[b] just before using.

REDUCING SOLUTION

Hydroquinone ....1.0 gm
Formalin, 37%-40% ....5.0 ml
Distilled water ....100.0 ml

1% GOLD CHLORIDE SOLUTION (Ch. 3)

2% OXALIC ACID SOLUTION (Ch. 3)

5% SODIUM THIOSULFATE (HYPO) SOLUTION (Ch. 3)

ANILINE BLUE SOLUTION

Aniline blue ....0.1 gm
Oxalic acid ....2.0 gm
Phosphomolybdic acid ....2.0 gm
Distilled water ....300.0 ml

PROCEDURE

1. Deparaffinize and hydrate to water.
2. Place in freshly prepared Protargol solution. Let stand at 37°C for 72 hours.
3. Rinse in 3 changes of distilled water.
4. Place in reducing solution for 10 minutes.
5. Rinse in 3 changes of distilled water.
6. Tone in 1% gold chloride solution for 10 minutes.
7. Rinse in 3 changes of distilled water.
8. Develop in 2% oxalic acid solution for 3 to 5 minutes.
9. Rinse in 3 changes of distilled water.
10. Treat with 5% sodium thiosulfate solution for 5 minutes.
11. Rinse in distilled water.
12. Counterstain with aniline blue solution for 1 to 5 minutes.

AFIP Laboratory Methods in Histotechnology

13.   Dehydrate and clear through 95% ethyl alcohol, absolute ethyl alcohol, and xylene, 2 changes each, for 2 minutes each.
14.   Mount with resinous medium.

RESULTS   (See Fig. 14–4, page 106).

Nerve fibers, myelinated and non-myelinated,
 and neurofibrils ....black
Background ....blue
Nuclei ....black

[a]Proteinate argenate can be obtained from Roboz Surgical Instruments Company Washington, DC.

[b]Copper shot can be obtained from North Strong Scientific, Rockville, MD.

REFERENCE
    Luna LG. Further studies of Bodian's technique. *Am J Med Technol.* 1964;30:355.

HOLMES METHOD FOR NERVE CELLS AND FIBERS

FIXATION: 10% buffered neutral formalin.

SECTIONS: Paraffin, 6 micrometers.

SOLUTIONS

20% SILVER NITRATE SOLUTION (Ch. 3)

1% SILVER NITRATE SOLUTION (Ch. 3)

10% PYRIDINE SOLUTION (Ch. 3)

0.2% GOLD CHLORIDE SOLUTION (Ch. 3)

2% OXALIC ACID SOLUTION (Ch. 3)

5% SODIUM THIOSULFATE (HYPO) SOLUTION (Ch. 3)

BORIC ACID BUFFER SOLUTION

Boric acid	12.4 gm
Distilled water	1000.0 ml

BORAX BUFFER SOLUTION

Sodium borate (Borax), tetra,	19.0 gm
Distilled water	1000.0 ml

IMPREGNATING SOLUTION

Boric acid buffer solution	55.0 ml
Borax buffer solution	45.0 ml
Distilled water	394.0 ml
Silver nitrate, 1%	1.0 ml
Pyridine, 10%	5.0 ml

REDUCING SOLUTION

Hydroquinone	1.0 gm
Sodium sulfite, crystals	10.0 gm
Distilled water	100.0 ml

PROCEDURE
1. Deparaffinize and hydrate to distilled water.
2. Place in 20% silver nitrate solution for 2 hours.
3. Rinse in 3 changes of distilled water, 3 minutes each.

4. Place in impregnating solution, in a covered staining dish, and leave in 37°C oven overnight.
5. Remove from oven, drain, and place in a clean dish.
6. Wash gently in running tap water for 2 minutes.
7. Rinse in distilled water.
8. Tone in gold chloride solution for 3 minutes.
9. Rinse quickly in distilled water.
10. Develop in oxalic acid solution for 3 to 5 minutes. Examine microscopically; allow to remain wet with the oxalic acid solution until axons are thoroughly blue black.
11. Rinse in distilled water.
12. Place in sodium thiosulfate for 5 minutes.
13. Wash in running tap water for 5 minutes.
14. Dehydrate and clear through 95% ethyl alcohol, absolute ethyl alcohol, and xylene, 2 changes each, for 2 minutes each.
15. Mount with resinous medium.

RESULTS

Axons (axis cylinders) .... black
Nerves and nerve endings .... black
Background .... gray to pink

REFERENCE

Holmes W. Silver staining of nerve axons in paraffin sections. *Anat Rec.* 1943;86:157.

LUXOL FAST BLUE (KLÜVER-BARRERA) METHOD FOR MYELIN AND NERVE CELLS

FIXATION: 10% buffered neutral formalin.

SECTIONS: Paraffin, 15 to 20 micrometers.

SOLUTIONS

0.1% LUXOL FAST BLUE SOLUTION

Luxol fast blue, MBS ....0.1 gm
Ethyl alcohol, 95% ....100.0 ml

Dissolve the dye in the alcohol. Add 0.5 ml of 10% acetic acid to each 100.0 ml of solution. Solution remains stable for months.

0.1% CRESYL ECHT VIOLET SOLUTION

Cresyl echt violet (cresyl fast violet) ....0.1 gm
Distilled water ....100.0 ml

Just before using, add 15 drops of 10% glacial acetic acid. Filter.

0.05% LITHIUM CARBONATE SOLUTION

Lithium carbonate ....0.05 gm
Distilled water ....100.0 ml

70% ETHYL ALCOHOL

PROCEDURE
1. Deparaffinize and hydrate to 95% ethyl alcohol.
2. Leave in luxol fast blue solution in 56°C oven overnight.
3. Rinse off excess stain with 95% ethyl alcohol.
4. Rinse in distilled water.
5. Differentiate the slides singly in the lithium carbonate solution for 30 seconds.
6. Continue differentiation in the 70% ethyl alcohol until the gray matter is clear and the white matter sharply defined.
7. Check microscopically. Repeat the differentiation if necessary, starting at step 5.
8. When differentiation is complete, place in distilled water.
9. When all slides have been collected in distilled water, add fresh distilled water.
10. Counterstain in the cresyl echt violet solution for 6 minutes. Optional counter stains include hematoxylin and eosin and the periodic acid-Schiff procedures.
11. Rinse in 2 changes of 95% ethyl alcohol.
12. Continue the dehydration through 2 changes of absolute ethyl alcohol and xylene, 2 changes each, for 2 minutes each.
13. Mount with resinous medium.

RESULTS   (See Fig. 14–5, page 106).

Myelin, including phospholipids ....blue to green
Cells and cell products ....pink to violet

The luxol fast blue procedure works well when combined with other procedures, as the Bodian method.

REFERENCE

Klüver H, Barrera E. A method for the combined staining of cells and fibers in the nervous system. *J Neuropathol Exp Neurol.* 1953;12:400.

WOELCKE'S MYELIN SHEATH PROCEDURE

FIXATION: 10% buffered neutral formalin.

SECTIONS: Paraffin, 20 micrometers.

SOLUTIONS

2.5% FERRIC AMMONIUM SULFATE SOLUTION (Ch. 3)

10% ALCOHOLIC HEMATOXYLIN STOCK SOLUTION (Ch. 3)

SATURATED LITHIUM CARBONATE SOLUTION

Lithium carbonate .... 1.54 gm
Distilled water .... 99.0 ml

HEMATOXYLIN WORKING SOLUTION

Mix the following ingredients in the order listed:
Distilled water .... 45.0 ml
Hematoxylin, alcoholic, 10% stock, filtered .... 10.0 ml
Lithium carbonate, saturated, filtered .... 7.0 ml
Distilled water .... 45.0 ml

It is essential to mix the ingredients in the order given. DO NOT SHAKE.

PROCEDURE

1. Deparaffinize and hydrate to distilled water.
2. Place in 2.5% ferric ammonium sulfate overnight.
3. Rinse in 2 changes of distilled water.
4. Stain in hematoxylin working solution for 2 hours.
5. Differentiate in 80% ethyl alcohol until background is clear.
6. Dehydrate and clear through 95% ethyl alcohol, absolute ethyl alcohol, and xylene, 2 changes each for 2 minutes each.
7. Mount with resinous medium.

RESULTS

Myelin sheaths, nuclei .... black
Glial cells .... black
Background .... clear

HIRSCH-PEIFFER METHOD FOR METACHROMATIC LEUCODYSTROPHY

FIXATION: 10% buffered neutral formalin.

SECTIONS: Paraffin, 12 to 20 micrometers.

SOLUTIONS

0.04% CRESYL VIOLET V STOCK SOLUTION

Cresyl violet V ....0.04 gm
Distilled water ....85.0 ml
Acetic acid, glacial ....15.0 ml

15% TRIETHANOLAMINE SOLUTION

Triethanolamine ....15.0 ml
Distilled water ....85.0 ml

CRESYL VIOLET-TRIETHANOLAMINE WORKING SOLUTION

Combine equal parts of cresyl violet V stock and 15% triethanolamine, as 100 ml each.

PROCEDURE

1. Deparaffinize and hydrate to distilled water.
2. Preheat cresyl violet-triethanolamine working solution in 60°C oven for 1 hour.
3. Stain in preheated cresyl violet-triethanolamine solution in a 60°C oven for 10 minutes.
4. Remove from oven. Cool to room temperature (20 to 25 minutes).
5. Transfer to distilled water.
6. Rinse in distilled water, 2 changes, for 5 minutes each.
7. Mount with glycerin jelly.

RESULTS (See Fig. 14–6, page 106).

Abnormal sulfatides ....brown
Other tissue structures ....blue to brown

---

REFERENCE
Hirsch V, Peiffer J. A histochemical study of the prelipid in metachromatic degenerative products in leucodystrophy. In: Cumings JN, ed. *Cerebral Lipidoses*. Oxford, England: Blackwells; 1957:68-76.

PHOSPHOTUNGSTIC ACID HEMATOXYLIN PROCEDURE

FIXATION: 10% buffered neutral formalin.

SECTIONS: Paraffin, 6 micrometers.

SOLUTIONS

PHOSPHOTUNGSTIC ACID HEMATOXYLIN SOLUTION

Hematoxylin .... 1.0 gm
Phosphotungstic acid .... 20.0 gm
Distilled water .... 100.0 ml

Dissolve the solid ingredients in portions of the distilled water. The hematoxylin will dissolve more readily with the aid of heat. When cool, it can be combined with the phosphotungstic acid and water mixture. No preservatives are necessary. Ripening ordinarily requires several weeks, but the addition of 0.2 gm of potassium permanganate will ripen the stain immediately. An alternative method for the immediate ripening is the use of 20 ml of freshly prepared 1% potassium permanganate solution.

0.25% POTASSIUM PERMANGANATE SOLUTION (Ch. 3)

LUGOL'S IODINE SOLUTION (Ch. 3)

5% OXALIC ACID SOLUTION (Ch. 3)

2.5% POTASSIUM DICHROMATE STOCK SOLUTION (Ch. 3)

POTASSIUM DICHROMATE WORKING SOLUTION

Potassium dichromate, 2.5% .... 95.0 ml
Acetic acid, glacial .... 5.0 ml

PROCEDURE

1. Deparaffinize and hydrate to distilled water.
2. Oxidize sections with potassium dichromate working solution overnight.
3. Wash gently in running tap water for 15 minutes.
4. Place in Lugol's iodine solution for 15 minutes.
5. Place in 95% alcohol for 1 hour to remove iodine. The brown color of the iodine is removed by several changes of 95% alcohol.
6. Rinse rapidly in 3 changes of distilled water.
7. Oxidize in 0.25% potassium permanganate for 5 minutes.
8. Rinse rapidly in 3 changes of distilled water.
9. Place in 5% oxalic acid for 5 minutes.
10. Rinse rapidly in 3 changes of distilled water.
11. Stain in phosphotungstic acid hematoxylin solution overnight.
12. Rinse in 95% alcohol to remove excess stain.

13. Dehydrate quickly with 3 changes of absolute alcohol.
14. Clear with xylene, 3 changes, for 3 minutes each.
15. Mount with resinous medium.

RESULTS   (See Fig. 14–7, page 107).

Nuclei, myelin sheaths, and glial cell processes ....blue

Cytoplasm ....pink

PENFIELD'S COMBINED METHOD FOR OLIGODENDROGLIA AND MICROGLIA

FIXATION: 10% buffered neutral formalin, formalin ammonium bromide.

SECTIONS: Frozen, 15 to 20 micrometers.

SOLUTIONS

FORMALIN AMMONIUM BROMIDE SOLUTION
Formaldehyde, 37% - 40% .... 15.0 ml
Ammonium bromide .... 2.0 gm
Distilled water .... 85.0 ml

5% HYDROBROMIC ACID SOLUTION (Ch. 3)

5% SODIUM CARBONATE SOLUTION (Ch. 3)

10% SILVER NITRATE SOLUTION (Ch. 3)

CONCENTRATED AMMONIUM HYDROXIDE (AMMONIA)

HORTEGA'S SILVER CARBONATE SOLUTION
Silver nitrate, 10% aqueous .... 5.0 ml
Sodium carbonate, 5% aqueous .... 20.0 ml

Add 28% ammonium hydroxide, drop by drop. Shake vigorously, adding sufficient quantities of ammonium hydroxide to dissolve the precipitate which forms. Add distilled water to make 75.0 ml.

1% FORMALIN SOLUTION (Ch. 3)

1% GOLD CHLORIDE STOCK SOLUTION (Ch. 3)

5% SODIUM THIOSULFATE (HYPO) SOLUTION (Ch. 3)

PROCEDURE
1. Place formalin-fixed tissues in formalin ammonium bromide for 3 to 5 days.
2. Mount sections on clean premarked slides. Dry thoroughly.
3. Place in distilled water to which has been added 10 to 15 drops of concentrated ammonium hydroxide. Leave overnight to remove traces of formalin.
4. Transfer to the hydrobromic acid solution. Place in 37°C oven for 1 hour.
5. Remove from oven and wash in 3 changes of distilled water.
6. Treat with sodium carbonate solution for 1 hour. Sections may be left in sodium carbonate solution without harmful effect.

7. Pour on the silver carbonate solution. Allow to react for 3 to 5 minutes. Check microscopically for the impregnation of the glial cells and their processes, wiping the back of the slide before placing it on the stage of the microscope. Treat again with silver carbonate solution if necessary.
8. Place in 1% formalin solution until sections are a uniform gray. Agitate gently.
9. Rinse thoroughly with distilled water.
10. Tone with the gold chloride solution until sections are blue-gray.
11. Rinse thoroughly with distilled water.
12. Fix with the sodium thiosulfate solution for 30 to 45 seconds.
13. Rinse with distilled water.
14. Dehydrate and clear through 95% ethyl alcohol, absolute ethyl alcohol, and xylene, 2 changes each, for 2 minutes each.
15. Mount with resinous medium.

RESULTS

Oligodendrocytes and microglia ....black
Background ....brown to yellow

REFERENCE

Penfield W. A method of staining oligodendroglia and microglia (combined method). *Am J Pathol.* 1928;4:153.

HOLZER'S METHOD FOR GLIAL FIBERS

FIXATION: 10% buffered neutral formalin or formol alcohol.

SECTIONS: Paraffin, 6 micrometers.

SOLUTIONS

PHOSPHOMOLYBDIC-ALCOHOL SOLUTION

Phosphomolybdic acid, 0.5% ....50.0 ml
Ethyl alcohol, 95% ....100.0 ml

Prepare fresh.

ABSOLUTE ALCOHOL-CHLOROFORM SOLUTION

Ethyl alcohol, 100% ....40.0 ml
Chloroform ....160.0 ml

Avoid inhaling the chloroform vapors by ensuring adequate ventilation.

CRYSTAL VIOLET SOLUTION

Crystal violet ....5.0 gm
Ethyl alcohol, 100% ....20.0 ml
Chloroform ....80.0 ml

POTASSIUM BROMIDE SOLUTION

Potassium bromide ....10.0 gm
Distilled water ....100.0 ml

It is economical to prepare 1000 ml of this solution at one time, hence 100 gm of potassium bromide in 1000 ml of distilled water.

DIFFERENTIATING SOLUTION

Aniline ....120.0 ml
Chloroform ....180.0 ml
Ammonium hydroxide, 28% ....20 drops

Avoid contact to the skin when using aniline.

PROCEDURE

1. Deparaffinize and hydrate to distilled water.
2. Place in phosphomolybdic alcohol solution for 3 minutes.
3. Drain.
4. Pour on alcohol-chloroform solution. Allow to remain until the sections become translucent.
5. Place on a staining rack and flood sections with the crystal violet solution for 30 seconds. Blot dry. If a precipitate of the crystal violet forms on the sections, it can be removed with undiluted aniline.
6. Return slides to the staining rack.
7. Flood sections with the potassium bromide solution for 1 minute. Blot dry.
8. Place in the differentiating solution for 30 seconds. If the slides are overdifferentiated, restain.

9. Rinse and clear in several changes of xylene. Check the slides microscopically after the first exchange of xylene.
10. Mount with resinous mounting medium.

RESULTS   (See Fig. 14–8, page 107).

Glial cells and fibers ....deep violet

Background ....pale violet

REFERENCE

Holzer W. Uber eine neue methode der gliofaser-farbung. *Zges Neuro Psychiat.* 1921;69:354.

CAJAL'S GOLD SUBLIMATE METHOD FOR ASTROCYTES

FIXATION: Formalin ammonium bromide.

SECTIONS: Frozen, 15 to 30 micrometers.

SOLUTIONS

FORMALIN AMMONIUM BROMIDE SOLUTION

Formaldehyde, 37% - 40%	15.0 ml
Ammonium bromide	2.0 gm
Distilled water	85.0 ml

CAJAL'S GOLD SUBLIMATE SOLUTION

Mercuric bichloride crystals	0.5 gm
Brown gold chloride, 1% aqueous	6.0 ml
Distilled water	35.0 ml

Store in brown bottle.

5% SODIUM THIOSULFATE (HYPO) SOLUTION (Ch. 3)

HORTEGA'S CARBOL-XYLENE CREOSOTE MIXTURE

Creosote	10.0 ml
Phenol crystals, melted	10.0 ml
Xylene	80.0 ml

PROCEDURE

1. Collect frozen sections in distilled water.
2. Place sections flat in freshly prepared gold chloride sublimate solution for 4 to 6 hours, in a dark place at room temperature.
3. Check a sample section microscopically when the section has turned purple.
4. Wash in distilled water for 5 to 10 minutes.
5. Place in sodium thiosulfate solution for 5 to 10 minutes.
6. Wash well in several changes of distilled water.
7. Float individual sections onto clean glass slides.
8. Air dry.
9. Start to dehydrate with 95% ethyl alcohol.
10. Clear in carbol-xylene creosote mixture or dehydrate and complete clearing by using 2 changes each of 95% ethyl alcohol, absolute ethyl alcohol, and xylene for 2 minutes each.
11. Mount with resinous medium.

RESULTS (See Fig. 14–9, page 107).

Astrocytes and their processes	black
Nerve cells	pale red
Nerve fibers	unstained
Background	clear to pale brown-purple

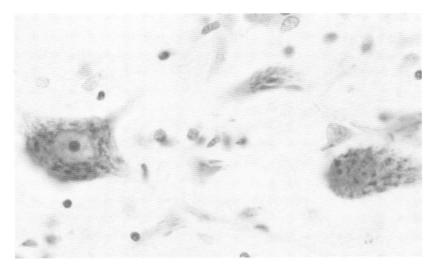

Fig. 14–1.
Cresyl violet.
Brain. Neuron with
Nissl bodies.

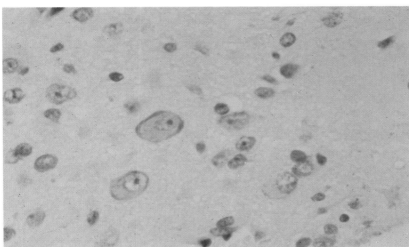

Fig. 14–2.
Gallocyanin.
Ganglioglioma.
Nissl substance in
ganglion cells
stains blue.

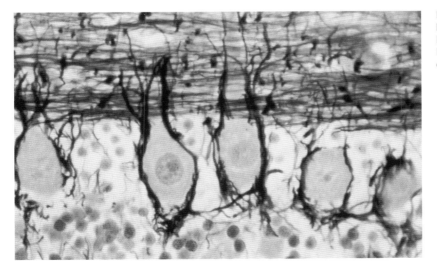

Fig. 14–3.
Modified
Bielschowsky.
Brain. Purkinje
cells with fibers.

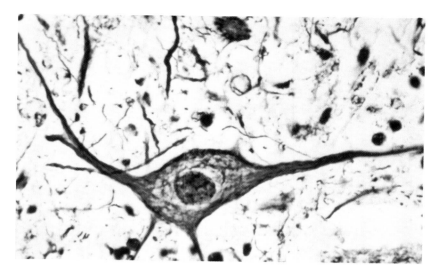

Fig. 14-4. Bodian. Brain. Neuron and processes.

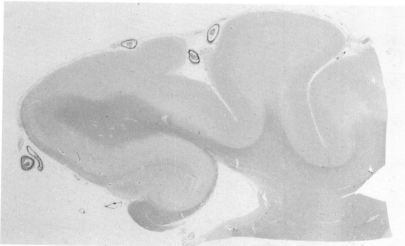

Fig. 14–5. Luxol fast blue with PAS. Brain. White matter stains blue.

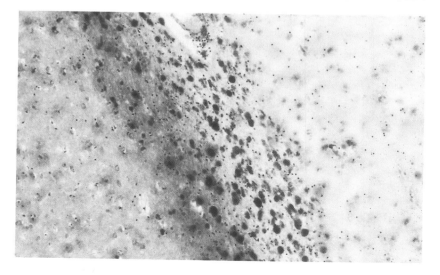

Fig. 14–6. Hirsch-Peiffer. Brain. Metachromatic leucodystrophy.

AFIP Laboratory Methods in Histotechnology

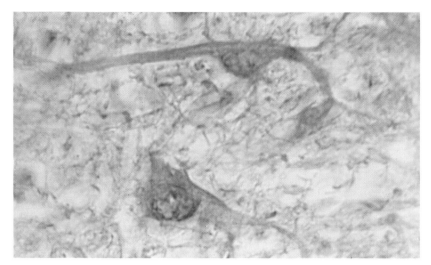

Fig.14-7.
PTAH. Brain.
Fibrillary
astrocytes.

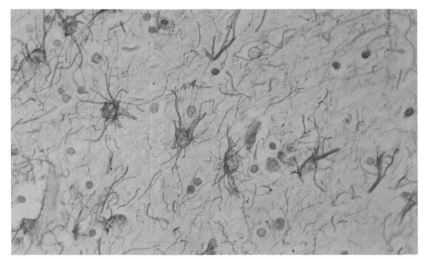

Fig. 14-8.
Holzer. Brain.
Fibrillary
astrocytes.

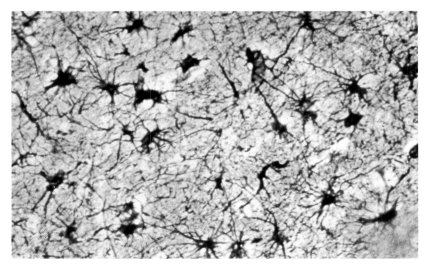

Fig. 14-9.
Cajal. Brain.
Astrocytes.

CHAPTER 15

OCULAR HISTOTECHNOLOGY

Peter V. Emanuele

The histologic preparation of whole eye specimens requires several technical modifications. The emphasis in this chapter will be on human eyes, but the recommendations can also be applied to equally large vertebrate eyes.

FIXATION

Ten percent buffered neutral formalin is recommended over fixatives containing mercuric chloride, chromates, or picric acid. The entire eye should be fixed without incisions, holes, or slices being made. The intact specimen will fix completely within 72 to 120 hours if an adequate volume, 1:15, of fixative is used.

DECALCIFICATION

Calcium salts or bone may be present in several sites within a shrunken blind eye. If there is extensive calcification or ossification inside the eye, the specimen cannot be cut properly. In such cases radiographs should be taken before cutting into an eyeball. (Another indication for radiographs is a history of an intraocular foreign body.) These radiographs then become a part of the permanent case record. The technologist should review the radiograph to determine the length of time needed for decalcification. We prefer the sodium citrate-formic acid procedure, which, though rather slow when compared to other acid solutions, will not overdecalcify or destroy the basophilic staining properties of the nuclei.

SODIUM CITRATE-FORMIC ACID DECALCIFICATION SOLUTION

SOLUTION A

Sodium citrate ....50.0 gm
Distilled water ....250.0 ml

SOLUTION B

Formic acid ....125.0 ml
Distilled water ....125.0 ml

Solution A and Solution B will remain stable for months. Store at room temperature.

WORKING SODIUM CITRATE-FORMIC ACID SOLUTION

Combine equal parts of Solution A and Solution B.

For eyes with minimal calcification, overnight treatment is recommended. The time can be extended up to 120 hours if calcium fills the specimen. Eyes with retinoblastoma should not be decalcified.

After decalcification the whole eye specimen should be thoroughly washed in running tap water for a minimum of 16 hours.

"GROSSING"

1. Orienting the eye

First determine whether it is a right or left eye. The identification of certain landmarks is of value (Fig. 15–1), especially the insertions of the oblique muscles and the long posterior ciliary arteries and nerves. The latter are almost always more prominent horizontally than in other meridians, and it is the tract of the long posterior ciliary artery and nerve (nasally) that is the most prominent. The superior oblique muscle has a tendinous insertion into the sclera, posterior to the temporal aspect of the superior rectus muscle. The inferior oblique muscle is the only extraocular muscle that inserts directly into the sclera by fleshy fibers; it has no tendon. This inferior oblique muscle inserts very near the horizontal meridian, temporal to the optic nerve and near the location of the macula.

Fig. 15–1
**External View of the Eye
Showing Muscles**

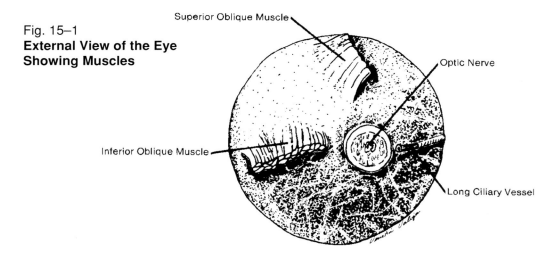

Superior Oblique Muscle

Optic Nerve

Inferior Oblique Muscle

Long Ciliary Vessel

2. Measuring the eye

Dimensions are listed by convention in the following order: for the whole eye, anteroposterior x horizontal x vertical; for the cornea, horizontal x vertical; for the optic nerve, the length attached to the globe. In the case of external markings, indicate meridian, anteroposterior location, and size.

3. Transillumination

Before an eye is opened, it should be transilluminated (held in front of a light bulb). The normal eye transmits light well except at the ciliary body/iris and at an optic nerve of significant length. Abnormal shadows should be mentioned in the gross description.

4. Opening the eye

Before opening the eyeball, a cross section of the optic nerve should be made. A central portion should be grossed so that the pupil and optic nerve (P-O) will appear in the final sections (Fig. 15–2). Despite these restrictions, the eye can still be opened in any meridian. The meridian chosen should add the most additional information to the P-O section. If neither clinical nor external findings nor the findings on transillumination suggest a meridian for opening the eye, then the eye should be opened horizontally to include the macular region in the P-O section.

Fig.15–2   **Sectioning the Eye**

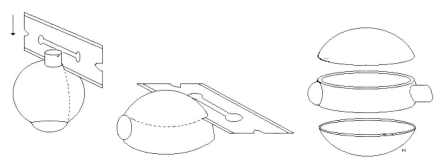

Having chosen a meridian, draw a red line on the sclera to follow with the razor knife. The red marks will dissolve during the processing steps which follow and for this reason are preferred to other color markings. With the eye held in one hand, the cornea down on a moistened paper towel, and the razor knife held between thumb and finger (Fig. 15 - 2) or in the blade handle, use a slow, sawing motion to make the first cut. Enter the eye from 1 to 2 mm to one side of the optic nerve. The cut should be directed to a point 1 mm central to the ipsilateral limbus. Complete about 1/3 of the first cut and then be sure that the cut is satisfactorily directed. By directing the blade to a point 1 mm posterior from the limbus, you will avoid the lens and the sawing motion of the razor knife will not dislocate the lens and distort the tissues of the anterior segment. If by chance the razor becomes engaged in the lens, complete the cut through the remaining tissues of the anterior segment by executing a guillotine-like motion, applying pressure straight down.

Make the second cut through the eye by placing the cut surface of the globe down on a moistened paper towel and cutting with the second edge of the razor knife. This can easily be accomplished by grasping the razor knife between the thumb and forefinger so that an equal length of thumbtip and fingertip extends beyond the blade, the length being equal to the desired thickness of the P-O segment. As with the first cut, proceed from the posterior pole anteriorly. With the second cut complete, there will be a P-O segment and two caps or calottes. A slice through either of the caps will yield a segment (Fig. 15–2). In the case of an intraocular foreign body, after opening the eye remove the foreign body by blunt dissection, measure it, and determine its magnetic properties. Use a disposable blade or an old microtome blade on these eyes.

The specimens selected for processing, usually the P-O and the cross section of the optic nerve, are then placed into metal cassettes with the identifying case numbers. If sections are desired from the caps or segments of the caps another cassette is required. The metal cassettes are then placed in a beaker containing 80% ethyl alcohol. At the end of the workday, the specimens are ready for processing.

Handling eyeballs containing synthetic intraocular lenses is the same as handling regular eyeballs without attempts to dissolve or remove them.

PROCESSING

AUTOMATIC

Grossed whole eye specimens, cross sections of the optic nerve, vortex vessels, segments, and caps can be processed automatically on an overnight schedule as described for routine tissues. The conventional 16-hour schedule applies. Peel-Away Embedding Compound should be used at the infiltration steps or at least for the embedding step.

MANUAL

In cases of large exenterated specimens containing the eyeball, eyelids, and orbital contents, the pathologist ensures that all orbital structures are aligned with the pupil and optic nerve. The size of these specimens necessitates manual processing. See Chapter 14, Neuropathological Histotechnology, for the manual processing schedule recommended for whole-mount brain specimens.

EMBEDDING

There are several considerations essential to the embedding of the grossed central portion of the eye: proper handling techniques, an embedding stand and metal pans, a heat lamp (a 1–amp, 150–watt flood lamp) and, to assist in the delicate handling of the specimen and the removal of entrapped air, a 6-inch angular forceps.

The overall dimension of the P-O segment, necessitates the use of the multiple embedding method and metal pans which are at least 1 inch deep. Cassettes, routinely used for other tissues, are usually not large enough for eyes.

The structures of the eye are delicate and require minimal handling by the technologist; the retina for example, can easily detach or be torn, and the lens dislocated by rough handling.

All entrapped air should be gently agitated out from the anterior and posterior chambers and from the delicate ocular layers.

Fig. 15–3 **Anatomy of the Eye**

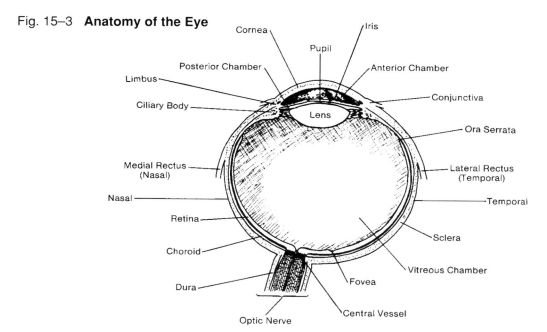

EMBEDDING PROCEDURE

1. Preheat the metal pan for 10 minutes, using a heat/flood lamp mounted approximately 8 inches above the pan. Fill embedding pan with filtered Peel Away paraffin.
2. Carefully open metal cassette containing the grossed specimen.
3. Remove the central portion (pupil and optic nerve [P-O]) from the cassette, using the forceps to pick it up. Hold any external connective tissue or muscle attachments. AVOID INSERTING THE FORCEPS IN THE SPECIMEN AS THIS CAN DAMAGE THE RETINA, LENS, ETC. (Figs. 15–3, 4)
4. Place the specimen in the molten paraffin with the identifying tag. (Fig. 15–5)
5. Agitate and rotate the specimen to remove any entrapped air.
6. Read the pathologist's gross description for embedding instructions.
7. Press the specimen to the bottom of the pan, holding the forceps in one hand and an ice cube in the other for cooling the bottom of the pan. (Fig. 15–6)
8. Allow the paraffin to cool until all of it is opaque. (Fig. 15–7)
9. Place pan containing the specimen in the freezer for 20 to 30 minutes. Avoid overcooling, which fractures the paraffin (fracture lines may be permanent in the retina and other delicate membranes.)
10. Release the paraffin from the pan.
11. Place the paraffin containing the specimen tissue side down on a paper towel. Then place it under the heat lamp, which is 6 to 8 inches above, and heat until pliable. (Fig. 15–8)
12. Make a block with a square or rectangular face, using a blunt knife, and remove the identification tag. (Fig. 15–9)
13. Place the block and the identification tag in a specimen box. (Fig. 15–10)
14. Write the identification number on the top and the sides of the box. Also indicate the type of specimen and the number of specimens enclosed.
15. Put the specimen box with the case folder. The specimen is ready for sectioning.

SECTIONING

EQUIPMENT AND MATERIALS NEEDED
—Microtome, rotary
—Microtome knife 185 mm
—Warming table, set at 38°C to 42°C
—Heated water bath (55°C to 56°C filled with distilled water)
—Rectangular glass dish (to serve as unheated water bath) filled with bubble-free distilled water and at room temperature
—Bowl for mounting blocks to block holder
—Bowl or dish for ice cubes
—Slides
—Rectangular strips of low-absorbency paper
—A 1-inch square of cotton
—Forceps, 6" long (angled and with a fine point)
—Gauze pads

PRELIMINARY PREPARATION
1.   Add to the heated and filled water bath 5 ml of a 5% solution of gelatin to which thymol has been added as a preservative.
2.   Using heat, mount the paraffin block for sectioning on a square block holder. Cool in a bowl of cold water.
3.   Set the microtome at 8 micrometers.

PROCEDURE
1.   Insert the block in the microtome. Be sure that the cornea and optic nerve are at the sides of the block. The cornea should never be at the top or bottom. Its placement away from either of these positions will result in a reduced number of artifacts and will help to ensure that surgical and trauma sites and the anterior and posterior poles will not be compressed.
2.   Trim the top, bottom, and sides of the block with a single-edged razor blade. Leave margins of paraffin on all sides. Avoid cutting into the opaque cornea. (Fig. 15–11)
3.   Note the pathologist's requests regarding sites of interest. Angling may be required to line up pupil, optic nerve, and lesions.
4.   Begin to "rough-cut," exercising care to avoid taking excessively thick slides. Microscopically examine a sample to ensure that the sections are near the sites of interest. Repeat this examination as often as necessary.

How to Flatten Rough-Cut Sections for Microscopic Examination.
Take a thick section from the knife edge using a camel's hair brush and float the section onto the surface of the rectangular dish containing the bubble-free distilled water. Pick the section up on a clean plain slide. Gradually lower the slide containing the thick slice into the heated water bath and allow it to spread. When it appears flat, pick the section up on the same slide. Wipe the undersurface and place on the microscope stage. Keeping the section moist, and using low or scanning power, lower the condenser and examine the section of eye microscopically. Discard the rough-cut slice.

5.   Place the square of cotton, which has been dipped into room-temperature water, over the exposed surface of the block. Soak the block for approximately 30 seconds. (Fig. 15–12) Avoid oversoaking.
6.   Clean the surface of the rectangular water bath and the heated water bath, using low-absorbency paper such as newspaper or pages from a telephone book. Discard the paper, which has picked up unwanted sections, dust, and other debris. (Fig. 15–13)
7.   Soak the block and exposed tissue so that the tissue will swell slightly. The moisture will be absorbed by the lens, hemorrhage, and exudate and will facilitate smooth sectioning. Rubbing the surface of the block with an ice cube and chilling the knife edge will facilitate smooth, wrinkle-free sections that form a ribbon.
8.   Turn the microtome wheel back, at least a quarter of a turn, to avoid a thick first section. Move the knife to a clean, sharp region. Never rough-cut and attempt ribboning at the same place on the knife.
9.   Proceed to take a ribbon which contains from 5 to 8, 8-micrometer sections. If a ribbon does not form, there are several reasons: dull knife, dirty knife edge, or top and bottom edges of the block are not parallel to the knife edge.
10. Replace the soaked cotton on the surface of the exposed tissue and block.

Repeat step 9.

11. Lift the ribbon from the knife using the fingers of one hand on the free end and a camel's hair brush on the knife end. (Fig. 15–14)

12. Carefully lower one end of the ribbon onto the room-temperature water in the rectangular dish and gradually lower the other end of the ribbon. (Fig. 15–15) Sections lowered in this manner will not have bubbles under them. Bubbles or entrapped air, if allowed to remain, reduce the section's adhesion to the glass slide and will produce small circular artifacts on microscopic examination of the stained slides.

13. Separate one section from the ribbon and place it on a clean slide. (Fig.15–16) Lower the glass slide containing the section onto the cleaned surface of the heated water bath.

14. Allow the section to spread. (Fig. 15–17) When all wrinkles are gone, orient the section and then lift it up and out of the water bath. (Fig. 15–18)

15. Check that the section matches the shape of the specimen in the block. (Fig. 15–19)

16. Label the slide with the case number. (Fig. 15–20)

17. Drain for several minutes, then place flat on the preset warming table and leave overnight. (Fig. 15–21)

18. The slides are ready for staining.

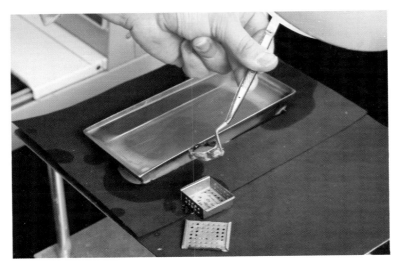

Fig. 15-4.
Removing P-O section from cassette, handling the external connective tissue. Note the metal pan and nearby lamp.

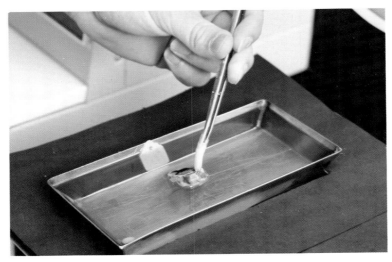

Fig. 15-5.
Placing specimen and identification tag in molten paraffin.

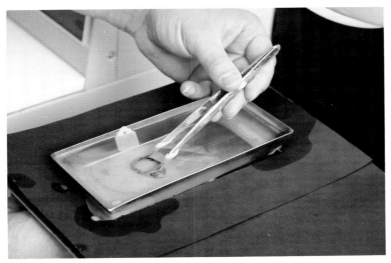

Fig. 15-6.
Orienting the specimen while cooling pan from below.

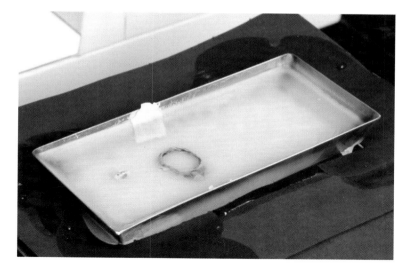

Fig. 15-7.
Cooling paraffin to
opacity.

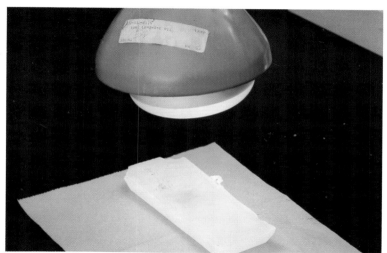

Fig. 15-8.
Softening paraffin with
lamp, tissue side down.

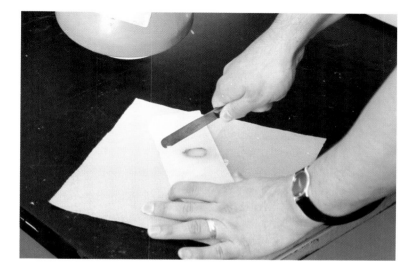

Fig. 15-9.
Preparing a block.

❖ Ocular Histotechnology

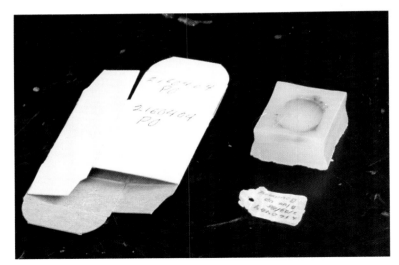

Fig. 15-10.
Specimen, tag, and box.

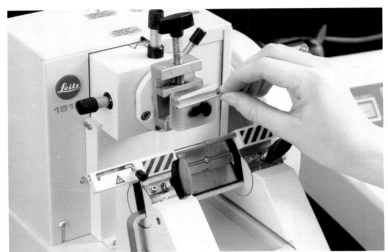

Fig. 15-11.
Trimming the block.

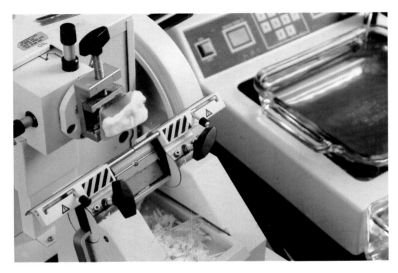

Fig. 15-12.
Soaking the block with
moist cotton.

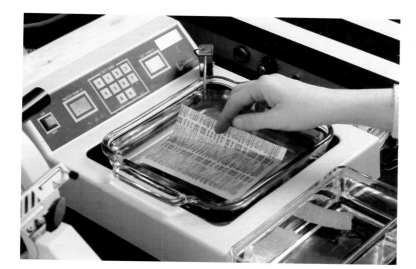

Fig. 15-13.
Cleaning the surface of
the heated water bath.

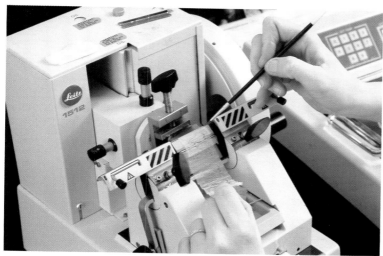

Fig. 15-14.
Lifting a ribbon.

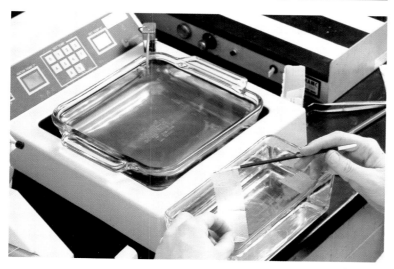

Fig. 15-15.
Placing a ribbon on the
room temperature water
bath.

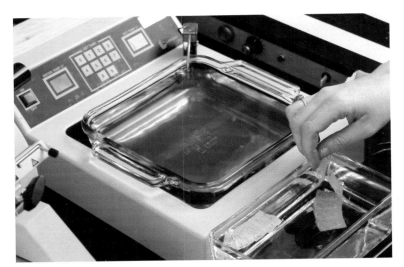

Fig. 15-16.
Picking up one
section from the room
temperature water bath.

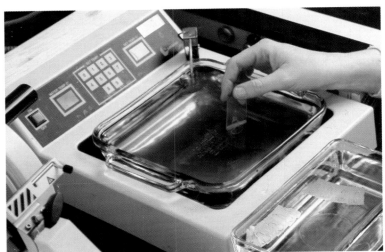

Fig. 15-17.
Spreading one section
on a water bath heated
to 55° –56°C.

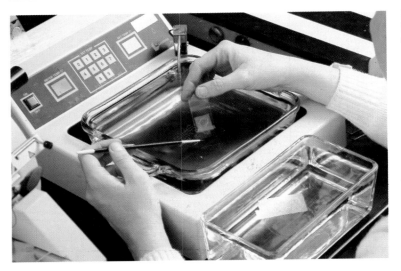

Fig. 15-18.
Lifting the wrinkle-free
section onto the slide.

AFIP Laboratory Methods in Histotechnology

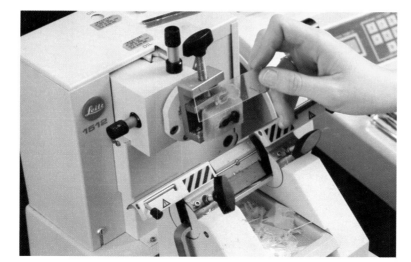

Fig. 15-19.
Matching the section on the slide with the surface of the block.

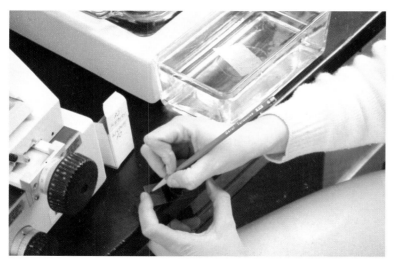

Fig. 15-20.
Labelling a slide with a hard lead pencil.

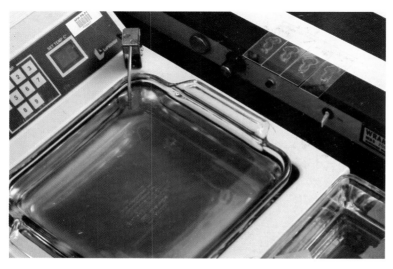

Fig. 15-21.
Drying on a warming table overnight.

CHAPTER 16

ANIMAL AND INSECT HISTOTECHNOLOGY

Debra A. McElroy

Processing, embedding, sectioning, and staining techniques for animal tissues are similar to the techniques for human tissues. This chapter describes techniques used for the preparation of animal and insect specimens.

FIXATION

The fixative of choice is 10% buffered neutral formalin. Bouin's or Zenker's may also be used.

PREPARATION AND PROCESSING OF INSECTS

Immediately following fixation, insect specimens should be soaked in 4% phenol solution (4 ml melted phenol in 96 ml 80% ethyl alcohol) for 24 hours to soften the chitinous exoskeletons and then processed as suggested in Table 16-1.

PREPARATION AND PROCESSING OF WORMS

After fixation, worms should be placed in two changes of N-butyl alcohol, 6 hours each, then infiltrated in a solution of equal parts of N-butyl alcohol and molten paraffin for 24 hours in an oven at 60°C, after which they are ready for embedding. N-butyl alcohol dehydrates and clears without excessive hardening.

PROCESSING AND EMBEDDING

Tissues from vertebrates like reptiles, fowl, rodents, and other small mammals should be processed separately as indicated in Table 16-2.

Certain tissues from the same species can be grouped together in cassettes for processing and embedding, whereas other tissues should be kept separate. For example, lung, heart, and muscle, pituitary gland and thyroid tissue, including parathyroid, should be embedded in separate blocks. As with human tissues, brain, spinal cord, nerve, eye, decalcified bone, testis, and bladder are generally processed and embedded separately. Muscles which are cut longitudinally are not usually embedded with those that are cut on cross section. Muscle specimens are embedded as close together as possible. Kidney, liver, spleen, and pancreas and portions of the digestive system can be processed and embedded together. The size of the specimens will determine how many can be combined in the same block.

SECTIONING

Following rough cutting, it is suggested that the exposed animal tissues be soaked in tepid water to facilitate ribboning. Alternative solutions for soaking very dry specimens are

(1) a solution of 50 ml of an ammoniated liquid detergent diluted with 10 ml of water, or (2) ammonium hydroxide solution diluted with an equal quantity of water.

For insects, following rough cutting, soak in tap water overnight then section at the desired thickness. Soaking in tap water softens very brittle specimens. Without soaking, the insects are virtually impossible to section without numerous artifacts.

H&E STAINING

1. Deparaffinize and hydrate in 2 changes each of xylene, absolute ethyl alcohol, and 95% ethyl alcohol for 3 minutes each.
2. Place in running tap water for 3 minutes.
3. Place in distilled water for 3 minutes.
4. Stain in Mayer's hematoxylin solution for 15 minutes.
5. Wash in warm tap water for 15 minutes.
6. Place in 80% alcohol for 3 minutes.
7. Counterstain in eosin/phloxine solution for 3 minutes. For fowl, one additional drop of glacial acetic acid is added just prior to use to ensure retention of counterstain.
8. Dehydrate and clear through 95% ethyl alcohol, absolute ethyl alcohol, and xylene, 2 changes each, 2 minutes each.
9. Mount using resinous medium.

RESULTS

Nuclei ....blue
Cytoplasm ....pink to red
Background ....pink to red

SPECIAL STAINING

There are no major modifications of the special stain procedures when applied to animal tissues.

REFERENCES

Coolidge BJ, Howard RM. *Animal histology procedures*. US Department of Health, Education and Welfare, NIH publication No. 90-275,1979.

Smith SG. A new embedding schedule for insect cytology. *Stain Technol*. 1949;14: 175.

Table 16–1

	INSECT PROCESSING SCHEDULE				
	WATER	ETHYL ALCOHOL	ALCOHOL	PHENOL	
Step (Dehydration and clearing)					
1	95.0 ml	5.0 ml			30 min
2	90.0 ml	10.0 ml			30 min
3	80.0 ml	20.0 ml			30 min
4	65.0 ml	35.0 ml			1 hr
5	50.0 ml	40.0 ml	10.0 ml		1 hr
6	30.0 ml	50.0 ml	20.0 ml		1 hr
7	15.0 ml	50.0 ml	35.0 ml	4.0 ml	24 hr
8	5.0 ml	40.0 ml	55.0 ml		1 hr
9		25.0 ml	75.0 ml		1 hr
10			100.0 ml	4.0 ml	1 hr
11			100.0 ml	4.0 ml	1 hr
12	(Infiltration) Paraffin, 3 changes, 3 hrs each.				

Table 16–2

VERTEBRATE PROCESSING SCHEDULES				
SOLUTIONS	REPTILES	FOWL	RODENT	PRIMATES CANINES FELINES
80% Isopropyl alcohol	30 min	30 min	1 hr	1 hr
80% Isopropyl alcohol	30 min	30 min	1 hr	1 hr
95% Isopropyl alcohol	30 min	30 min	1 hr	1 hr
95% Isopropyl alcohol	30 min	30 min	1 hr	1 hr
95% Isopropyl alcohol	30 min	30 min	1 hr	1 hr
100% Isopropyl alcohol	30 min	30 min	1 hr	1 hr
100% Isopropyl alcohol	30 min	30 min	1 hr	1 hr
100% Isopropyl alcohol	30 min	30 min	1 hr	1 hr
Xylene	30 min	30 min	1 hr	1 hr
Xylene	30 min	1 hr	1 hr	1 hr
Paraffin	30 min	40 min	40 min	1 hr
Paraffin	30 min	40 min	40 min	1 hr
Paraffin	30 min	40 min	40 min	1 hr

Each station has pressure/vacuum to accomplish the above schedules.

CHAPTER 17

CONNECTIVE TISSUE

Debra A. McElroy

Connective tissues consist of cells and extracellular fibers that are embedded in ground substance.

CELLS OF CONNECTIVE TISSUE: Fibroblasts, fat cells (adipocytes), mast cells, cartilage cells (chondrocytes), and bone cells (osteocytes).

FIBERS OF CONNECTIVE TISSUE: Collagen, reticulum, and elastin.

Collagen. Collagen is the predominant fiber and is easily demonstrated with routine hematoxylin-eosin stains. Selected special stains (e.g., Masson's trichrome and Gomori's trichrome) are useful to distinguish collagen from muscle and other elements.

Reticulum. Reticulum fibers are highly branched, delicate argyrophilic fibers that stain with ammoniacal silver solutions (e.g., the Snook, Wilder, and Manuel methods.)

Elastin. Elastic fibers are demonstrated with iron hematoxylin, resorcin fuchsin, or aldehyde fuchsin. Verhoeff's procedure uses iron hematoxylin; Gomori's aldehyde fuchsin, an aldehyde fuchsin solution; and Hart's elastica procedure, a resorcin fuchsin solution.

GROUND SUBSTANCE: This includes the following: hyaluronic acid (see Chapter 18, Carbohydrates), chondroitin sulfate, and dermatin sulfate.

The aqueous phase of ground substance is the medium through which nutrients and wastes pass.

The procedures listed in this chapter will identify some of the structures listed above, as well as selected hematologic stains. The chapters on carbohydrates and lipids cover other procedures for specific connective tissue components.

MODIFIED RUSSELL-MOVAT PENTACHROME METHOD

FIXATIVE: 10% buffered neutral formalin.

SECTIONS: Paraffin, 6 micrometers.

SOLUTIONS

10% ALCOHOLIC HEMATOXYLIN SOLUTION (Ch. 3)

10% FERRIC CHLORIDE SOLUTION (Ch. 3)

VERHOEFF'S IODINE SOLUTION

Iodine	2.0 gm
Potassium iodide	4.0 gm
Distilled water	100.0 ml

Mix the 2 grams of iodine and the 4 grams of iodide in a flask. Shake vigorously. Then gradually add the distilled water, 20 ml at a time.

VERHOEFF'S ELASTIC STAIN WORKING SOLUTION

Alcoholic hematoxylin, 10%	25.0 ml
Alcohol, 100% ethyl	25.0 ml
Ferric chloride, 10%	25.0 ml

Mix well, then add:

Verhoeff's iodine solution	25.0 ml

2% FERRIC CHLORIDE DIFFERENTIATING SOLUTION

Ferric chloride, 10%	20.0 ml
Distilled water	80.0 ml

5% SODIUM THIOSULFATE (HYPO) SOLUTION (Ch. 3)

3% GLACIAL ACETIC ACID SOLUTION (Ch. 3)

1% ALCIAN BLUE SOLUTION

Alcian blue, 8GS	1.0 gm
Distilled water	97.0 ml
Acetic acid, glacial	3.0 ml

CROCEIN SCARLET-ACID FUCHSIN STOCK SOLUTION

Solution A

Crocein scarlet	0.1 gm
Distilled water	99.5 ml
Acetic acid, glacial	0.5 ml

Solution B

        Acid fuchsin ....0.1 gm

        Distilled water..99.5 ml

        Acetic acid, glacial ....0.5 ml

CROCEIN SCARLET-ACID FUCHSIN WORKING SOLUTION

        Solution A..80.0 ml

        Solution B..20.0 ml

1% GLACIAL ACETIC ACID SOLUTION (Ch. 3)

5% PHOSPHOTUNGSTIC ACID SOLUTION (Ch. 3)

ALCOHOLIC SAFFRON SOLUTION

        Saffron du Gatinais[a]. ....6.0 gm

        Alcohol, absolute, ...100.0 ml

Shake well. Saffron will not completely dissolve. Let sit for 24 hours. To use, decant without disturbing the sediment. Save solution after use.

PROCEDURE

1. Deparaffinize and hydrate to distilled water.
2. Stain in Verhoeff's elastic stain working solution for 15 to 30 minutes.[b]
3. Wash in running lukewarm tap water for 20 minutes.
4. Place in distilled water.
5. Differentiate in 2% ferric chloride solution.[c] Check microscopically. When elastic fibers are sharply defined, the background appears gray. Rinse in distilled water to stop the reaction.
6. Place in 5% sodium thiosulfate solution for 1 minute.
7. Wash in tap water for 5 minutes.
8. Place in 3% glacial acetic acid solution for 3 minutes.
9. Place directly in 1% alcian blue solution for 15 to 30 minutes or until the mucins are stained blue and the muscle clears.
10. Rinse thoroughly in running warm tap water for 10 minutes.
11. Rinse in distilled water.
12. Stain in Crocein scarlet-acid fuchsin solution for 2 minutes.
13. Rinse in several changes of distilled water.
14. Rinse quickly in 1% acetic acid solution.
15. Place in 5% phosphotungstic acid solution for 2 changes, 2-5 minutes each. Check microscopically.[d]
16. Rinse in 1% acetic acid solution.
17. Dehydrate slides in 3 changes of absolute ethyl alcohol.
18. Stain in alcoholic saffron solution for 15 minutes.
19. Rinse slides in 3 changes of absolute ethyl alcohol and clear in 2 changes of xylene.
20. Mount with resinous medium.

RESULTS   (See Fig. 17–1, page 147).

Nuclei .... black
Elastic fibers .... black
Collagen .... yellow
Ground substance and mucins .... blue to green
Muscle .... red
Fibrinoid .... intense red

[a]Avoid exposure of saffron solution to water. Keep Coplin jar and stock solutions covered at all times to prevent moisture contamination.

[b]The staining of the elastic fibers before the mucosubstances has shortened the overall staining time and improved the quality.

[c]At step 5, differentiate the slides in 2% ferric chloride solution at 15 second intervals. Between the intervals, drain off the residual ferric chloride solution and dip slide in distilled water to check microscopically. Continue differentiation until the elastic fibers of larger arteries can be distinguished from the muscle.

[d]Check microscopically to determine if connective tissue is clear. Stop differentiation before elastic fibers are destained.

REFERENCES

Movat HZ. Demonstration of all connective tissue elements in a single section. *Arch Path.* 1955;60:289.

Russell K. Pentachrome stain modification. *Arch Path.* 1972;94:187.

GOMORI'S ONE-STEP TRICHROME STAIN

FIXATION: Any well-fixed tissue, including alcohol-fixed smears.

SECTIONS: Paraffin, 6 micrometers.

SOLUTIONS

BOUIN'S FIXATIVE SOLUTION (Ch. 3)

IRON HEMATOXYLIN WORKING SOLUTION[a], WEIGERT'S (Ch. 3)

GOMORI'S TRICHROME STAIN

Chromotrope 2R ....0.6 gm
Light green[b] ....0.3 gm
Glacial acetic acid ....1.0 ml
Phosphotungstic acid..0.8 gm
Distilled water...100.0 ml

1% GLACIAL ACETIC ACID SOLUTION (Ch. 3)

PROCEDURE
1. Deparaffinize and hydrate to distilled water.
2. Place in Bouin's fixative in oven at 56°C for one hour.[c]
3. Wash well in running water until sections are clear.
4. Stain in Weigert's iron hematoxylin working solution for 10 minutes.
5. Rinse in tap water.
6. Stain in Gomori's trichrome stain for 15 to 20 minutes.
7. Rinse in 1% acetic acid.[d]
8. Rinse in distilled water.
9. Dehydrate and clear in 95% ethyl alcohol, absolute ethyl alcohol, and xylene, 2 changes each, 2 minutes each.
10. Mount with resinous medium.

RESULTS

Muscle fibers ....red
Collagen ....green
Nuclei...blue to black

[a]Gomori's chromium hematoxylin may be substituted for the Weigert's iron hematoxylin at step 4.

[b]Aniline blue can be substituted for the light green.

[c]Slides may be left in Bouin's solution overnight at room temperature.

[d]If sections are too red, differentiate in 100 ml of 1% acetic acid to which 0.7 gms of phosphotungstic acid has been added.

REFERENCE
Gomori GL. A rapid one-step trichrome. *Amer J Clin Path.* 1950;20:661.

MASSON'S TRICHROME STAIN

FIXATION: 10% buffered neutral formalin. Bouin's fixative.

SECTIONS: Paraffin, 6 micrometers.

SOLUTIONS

BOUIN'S FIXATIVE (Ch. 3)

IRON HEMATOXYLIN WORKING SOLUTION, WEIGERT'S (Ch. 3)

BIEBRICH SCARLET-ACID FUCHSIN SOLUTION

Biebrich scarlet, 1% aqueous ....90.0 ml
Acid fuchsin, 1% aqueous ....10.0 ml
Acetic acid, glacial ....1.0 ml

PHOSPHOMOLYBDIC-PHOSPHOTUNGSTIC ACID SOLUTION

Phosphomolybdic acid ....5.0 gm
Phosphotungstic acid ....5.0 gm
Distilled water...200.0 ml

ANILINE BLUE SOLUTION

Aniline blue ....2.5 gm
Acetic acid, glacial ....2.0 ml
Distilled water...100.0 ml

OR

LIGHT GREEN SOLUTION

Light green ....5.0 gm
Distilled water...250.0 ml
Glacial acetic acid ....2.0 ml

1% ACETIC ACID SOLUTION (Ch. 3)

PROCEDURE

1. Deparaffinize and hydrate to distilled water.
2. Treat with Bouin's fixative solution if sections are formalin fixed for 1 hour at 56°C *or* overnight at room temperature. Omit step if tissues were fixed in Bouin's solution initially.
3. Let stand for 10 minutes to cool.
4. Wash in running water until sections are clear. Rinse in distilled water.
5. Stain in Weigert's iron hematoxylin solution for 10 minutes.
6. Wash in running water for 10 minutes. Rinse in distilled water.
7. Stain in Biebrich scarlet-acid fuchsin solution for 15 minutes.[a] Save solution. Rinse in distilled water.

8. Differentiate in phosphomolybdic-phosphotungstic acid solution for 10 to 15 minutes. Check to see that collagen is not red.[b]

9. Counterstain in aniline blue solution for 5 to 10 minutes or light green solution for 1 minute. Save solution. Rinse in distilled water.

1Oa. If aniline blue solution is used, differentiate in 1% acetic water, 3 to 5 minutes.

1Ob. If light green solution is used, differentiate in 5% phosphotungstic acid solution for 15 minutes.

11. Dehydrate and clear through 95% ethyl alcohol, absolute ethyl alcohol, and xylene, 2 changes each, 2 minutes each.

12. Mount with resinous medium.

RESULTS (See Fig. 17–2, page 147).

Nuclei .... black
Muscle, cytoplasm, keratin .... red
Collagen .... blue or green

[a]For central nervous system sections, the staining times are different:

Step 7. Biebrich scarlet-acid fuchsin solution for 2 minutes.
Step 8. Phosphomolybdic-phosphotungstic acid solution for 10 to 30 minutes.
Step 9. Aniline blue solution for 15 to 20 minutes.

[b]Repeat differentiation in phosphomolybdic-phosphotungstic acid if collagen retains the red color from the Biebrich scarlet solution.

REFERENCE
Masson PJ. Trichrome stainings and their preliminary techniques. *J Tech Met.* 1929;12:75.

VERHOEFF'S ELASTIC STAIN

FIXATION: 10% buffered neutral formalin or any other well-fixed tissue.

SECTIONS: Paraffin, 6 micrometers.

SOLUTIONS

10% ALCOHOLIC HEMATOXYLIN SOLUTION (Ch. 3)

10% FERRIC CHLORIDE SOLUTION (Ch. 3)

VERHOEFF'S IODINE SOLUTION

Iodine ....2.0 gm
Potassium iodide ....4.0 gm
Distilled water...100.0 ml

Mix the crystals of iodine and the crystals of iodide in a flask. Shake vigorously. Then gradually add the distilled water, 20 ml at a time.

VERHOEFF'S ELASTIC STAIN WORKING SOLUTION

Alcoholic hematoxylin, 10% ....25.0 ml
Alcohol, 100% ethyl ....25.0 ml
Ferric chloride, 10% ....25.0 ml
Mix well, then add:
Verhoeff's iodine solution ....25.0 ml

2% FERRIC CHLORIDE DIFFERENTIATING SOLUTION

Ferric chloride, 10% ....20.0 ml
Distilled water...80.0 ml

VAN GIESON SOLUTION (Ch. 3)

5% SODIUM THIOSULFATE (HYPO) SOLUTION (Ch. 3)

PROCEDURE
1. Deparaffinize and hydrate to distilled water.
2. Stain in Verhoeff's elastic stain working solution for 15 minutes.
3. Wash in lukewarm running tap water for 20 minutes.
4. Place in distilled water.
5. Differentiate in 2% ferric chloride solution. Check microscopically.[a] Elastic fibers are black and sharply fined; the background is gray.
6. Place in 5% sodium thiosulfate solution for 1 minute.
7. Wash in tap water for 5 minutes.
8. Place in distilled water.
9. Counterstain in van Gieson solution for 1 minute.[b]

10. Dehydrate rapidly[c] through 95% ethyl alcohol (2 changes) and absolute ethyl alcohol (2 changes); clear in 2 changes of xylene.
11. Mount with resinous medium.

RESULTS

Elastic fibers ....black
Nuclei ....black
Collagen ....red
Other tissue structures..yellow

[a]Wipe the back of the slide. While wet with the 2% ferric chloride differentiation solution, check under low power. Elastic fibers in arterial walls should be black and the arterial wall muscle, gray.

[b]Do not leave in van Gieson solution for more than 1 minute. The picric acid component decolorizes the elastic fibers.

[c]Rinse rapidly in 95% ethyl alcohol to avoid decolorizing the van Gieson solution.

REFERENCE
Mallory FB. *Pathological Technique.* Philadelphia, PA: WB Saunders; 1942:170-171.

VAN GIESON'S PICRIC ACID AND ACID FUCHSIN STAIN

FIXATION: 10% buffered neutral formalin.

TECHNIQUE: Paraffin, 4 to 6 micrometers.

SOLUTIONS

IRON HEMATOXYLIN STOCK SOLUTION, WEIGERT'S (Ch. 3)

IRON HEMATOXYLIN WORKING SOLUTION, WEIGERT'S (Ch. 3)

1% AQUEOUS ACID FUCHSIN SOLUTION (Ch. 3)

SATURATED PICRIC ACID SOLUTION[a]

Picric acid	1.2 gm
Distilled water	100.0 ml

VAN GIESON STAIN

Acid fuchsin, 1% aqueous	5.0 ml
Picric acid solution, saturated	95.0 ml

PROCEDURE
1. Deparaffinize and hydrate to distilled water.
2. Stain in Weigert's hematoxylin working solution for 10 minutes.
3. Rinse in distilled water.
4. Stain in van Gieson solution for 1 to 3 minutes.
5. Dehydrate and clear through 95% ethyl alcohol, absolute ethyl alcohol, and xylene, 2 changes each, 2 minutes each.
6. Mount with resinous medium.

RESULTS

Collagen	red
Muscle	yellow
Cornified epithelium	yellow
Nuclei	black

[a]Avoid making a supersaturated solution by measuring the picric acid precisely.

REFERENCE
Mallory FB. *Pathological technique*. Philadelphia, PA: WB Saunders; 1938: 152-153.

MANUEL'S METHOD FOR RETICULUM

FIXATION: 10% buffered neutral formalin.

TECHNIQUE: Paraffin, 6 micrometers.

SOLUTIONS

1% URANIUM NITRATE SOLUTION (Ch. 3)

AMMONIACAL SILVER SOLUTION

Silver nitrate .... 100.0 gm
Distilled water .... 1000.0 ml
Mix thoroughly.
Remove 70 ml of the above 10% silver nitrate solution.
Set aside.
To the remaining 930 ml of the 10% silver nitrate solution,
Add:

Ammonium hydroxide, 28% .... 60.0 ml

Slowly add 50 ml of the reserved 70 ml silver nitrate solution. Add all or a portion of the 20 ml of silver nitrate solution which remains until the resulting solution becomes slightly cloudy. This can be stored in the refrigerator for several months.

1% FORMALIN SOLUTION (Ch. 3)

5% SODIUM THIOSULFATE (HYPO) SOLUTION (Ch. 3)

NUCLEAR FAST RED (KERNECHTROT) SOLUTION (Ch. 3)

PROCEDURE
1. Deparaffinize and hydrate to distilled water.
2. Sensitize in uranium nitrate solution, 2 minutes.
3. Dip quickly in running water.
4. Impregnate in ammoniacal silver solution for 1 minute.
5. Wash in running water, 2 or 3 quick dips, until no more white precipitate appears in the water.
6. Develop in formalin solution for 1 minute.
7. Wash in running water.
8. Tone in gold chloride solution for 1 minute.
9. Wash in running water.
10. Reduce in sodium thiosulfate solution for 1 minute.
11. Wash in running water.
12. Counterstain in nuclear fast red solution, 5 minutes.
13. Rinse in distilled water 3 changes.

14. Dehydrate and clear through 95% ethyl alcohol, absolute ethyl alcohol, and xylene, 2 changes each, 2 minutes each.
15. Mount with resinous medium.

RESULTS (See Fig. 17–3, page 147).

Reticulum ....black
Nuclei and background ....red

SNOOK'S METHOD FOR RETICULUM

FIXATION: 10% buffered neutral formalin.

SECTIONS: Paraffin, 6 micrometers.

SOLUTIONS

0.25% POTASSIUM PERMANGANATE SOLUTION (Ch. 3)

5% OXALIC ACID SOLUTION (Ch. 3)

1% URANIUM NITRATE SOLUTION (Ch. 3)

5% SILVER NITRATE SOLUTION (Ch. 3)

10% SODIUM HYDROXIDE SOLUTION (Ch. 3)

SNOOK'S AMMONIACAL SILVER SOLUTION[a]

Silver nitrate, 5% ....20.0 ml
Add:
Sodium hydroxide, 10% ....20 drops
While shaking add:

Ammonium hydroxide, concentrated, drop by drop until the solution clears and a few granules remain at the bottom of the cylinder. Filter and use immediately.

1% FORMALIN SOLUTION[a] (Ch. 3)

1% GOLD CHLORIDE SOLUTION (Ch. 3)

5% SODIUM THIOSULFATE (HYPO) SOLUTION (Ch. 3)

NUCLEAR FAST RED (KERNECHTROT) SOLUTION (Ch. 3)

PROCEDURE
1. Deparaffinize and hydrate to distilled water.
2. Oxidize in potassium permanganate solution for 5 minutes.
3. Wash in tap water.
4. Oxalic acid solution until sections are clear.
5. Wash in tap water, then place in distilled water.
6. Mordant in uranium nitrate solution for 5 seconds.
7. Wash in running water.
8. Ammoniacal silver solution for 1 minute.[b]
9. Dip in running water.

10. 1% formalin solution for 1 minute.
11. Wash in running water.
12. 1% gold chloride solution until sections are grayish black, 1 minute.
13. Wash in running water.
14. Sodium thiosulfate solution for 30 seconds to 1 minute.
15. Wash in running water.
16. Counterstain in nuclear fast red solution for 5 minutes.
17. Rinse in distilled water.
18. Dehydrate and clear through 95% ethyl alcohol, absolute ethyl alcohol, and xylene 2 changes, 2 minutes each.
19. Mount with resinous medium.

RESULTS

Reticulum fibers ....gray to black
Background ....pink to rose

[a]Replace solutions after every 10 or 12 slides.

[b]Use acid clean Coplin jars and paraffin coated forceps or Teflon forceps for steps 8 through 18, and for steps 8 to 15 carry slides through one at a time.

REFERENCE
Snook T. The guinea pig spleen; studies on the structure and connections of the venous sinuses. *Anat Rec.* 1944;89:413.

WILDER'S METHOD FOR RETICULUM

FIXATION: 10% buffered neutral formalin.

SECTIONS: Paraffin, 6 micrometers.

SOLUTIONS

10% PHOSPHOMOLYBDIC ACID SOLUTION (Ch. 3)

1% URANIUM NITRATE SOLUTION (Ch. 3)

10.2% SILVER NITRATE SOLUTION

Silver nitrate .... 10.2 gm
Distilled water .... 100.0 ml

3.1% SODIUM HYDROXIDE SOLUTION

Sodium hydroxide .... 3.1 gm
Distilled water .... 100.0 ml

AMMONIACAL SILVER SOLUTION[a]

Silver nitrate solution .... 5.0 ml
Add:
Ammonium hydroxide, concentrated drop by drop until the
precipitate which forms is almost dissolved.
Add:
Sodium hydroxide solution .... 5.0 ml
Solution will be precipitated again.
Add:
Ammonium hydroxide, concentrated, drop by drop until solution clears.
Make the solution up to 50.0 ml with distilled water.

REDUCING SOLUTION

Distilled water .... 50.0 ml
Formalin, neutral, 40% .... 0.5 ml
Uranium nitrate, 1% .... 1.5 ml

0.2% GOLD CHLORIDE SOLUTION (Ch. 3)

5% SODIUM THIOSULFATE (HYPO) SOLUTION (Ch. 3)

NUCLEAR FAST RED (KERNECHTROT) SOLUTION (Ch. 3)

PROCEDURE
1. Deparaffinize and hydrate to distilled water.
2. Oxidize in phosphomolybdic acid solution for 1 minute.

3. Rinse thoroughly in running water until all traces of the yellow solution disappear.
4. 1% uranium nitrate solution for 1 minute.
5. Rinse in distilled water for 10-20 seconds.
6. Ammoniacal silver solution for 1 minute.[a]
7. Dip very quickly in 95% alcohol.
8. Reducing solution for 1 minute.
9. Rinse in distilled water.
10. Tone in 0.2% gold chloride solution for 1 minute.[b]
11. Rinse in distilled water.
12. Sodium thiosulfate solution for 1 minute.
13. Wash in tap water.
14. Counterstain with nuclear fast red solution for 5 minutes.
15. Rinse well in distilled water.
16. Dehydrate and clear with 95% ethyl alcohol, absolute ethyl alcohol, and xylene, 2 changes each, 2 minutes each.
17. Mount with resinous medium.

RESULTS

Reticulum fibers .... black
Collagen .... rose
Other tissue elements .... red

[a]Approximately 5 to 7 slides may be passed through the ammoniacal silver solution after which the solution should be changed.

[b]Prolonged exposure to the gold chloride solution will overtone the reticulum fibers and they will appear red in the final slides.

REFERENCE
Wilder HC. An improved technic for silver impregnation of reticulum fibers. *Amer J Path.* 1935;11:817.

METHYL GREEN–PYRONIN METHOD FOR DNA & RNA
AFIP Modification

FIXATION: 10% buffered neutral formalin or Carnoy's fixative.

SECTIONS: Paraffin, 4 micrometers

SOLUTIONS
1% METHYL GREEN STOCK SOLUTION

Methyl green .... 1.0 gm
Distilled water .... 100.0 ml

Extract the impurity, methyl violet, from the solution, using the following procedure:

CHLOROFORM EXTRACTION

1. Pour 100 ml of 1% methyl green stock solution into a separatory funnel. Then add an equal volume of chloroform. Mix well.
2. Allow the extraction to continue for several hours or overnight, if possible.
3. Discard the discolored chloroform, at the bottom.
4. Repeat by adding equal amounts of chloroform until the chloroform is colorless. Usually, three changes, every three hours is sufficient to remove all impurities from the 1% methyl green stock solution. This solution is now ready for the preparation of the methyl green-pyronin working solution.

1% PYRONIN GS STOCK SOLUTION

Pyronin GS .... 1.0 gm
Distilled water .... 100.0 ml

Heat gently and stir frequently to dissolve the pyronin.

METHYL GREEN-PYRONIN WORKING SOLUTION

Methyl green, 1% solution,
    after extraction procedure .... 70.0 ml
Pyronin GS, 1% stock solution .... 30.0 ml

Adjust pH to exactly 4.8 using 1% sodium acetate solution. Allow to stand overnight before using. Do not filter.

1% SODIUM ACETATE SOLUTION

Sodium acetate .... 1.0 gm
Distilled water .... 100.0 ml

ACETONE

PROCEDURE
1. Deparaffinize and hydrate to distilled water.
2. Place in unfiltered methyl green-pyronin working solution for 2 minutes.
3. Blot slides with bibulous paper then air dry for 5 minutes.

4. Differentiate the slides individually in distilled water, 1 or 2 rapid dips. Check microscopically. If sections are too red, differentiate quickly in very cold (-5°C) 80% ethyl alcohol.
5. Start dehydration in acetone, 2 or 3 quick dips.
6. Complete dehydration and clearing in equal parts of acetone and xylene, and xylene, 2 changes each, 1 to 2 minutes each.
7. Mount using resinous medium.

RESULTS

Ribonucleic acid (RNA) ....red
Desoxyribonucleic acid (DNA) ....blue to blue green

REFERENCE
Kurnick NB. Histological staining with methyl-green-pyronin. *Stain Technol.* 1952;27:233.

LUNA'S METHOD FOR MAST CELLS

FIXATION: 10% buffered neutral formalin.

SECTIONS: Paraffin, 6 micrometers.

SOLUTIONS

ALDEHYDE FUCHSIN SOLUTION (Ch. 3)

IRON HEMATOXYLIN WORKING SOLUTION, WEIGERT'S (Ch. 3)

METHYL ORANGE SOLUTION

Methyl orange .... 0.25 gm
Alcohol, 95% ethyl .... 100.0 ml

PROCEDURE

1. Deparaffinize and hydrate to 95% alcohol.
2. Stain in aldehyde fuchsin solution for 30 minutes.
3. Rinse in 95% alcohol.
4. Stain in Weigert's iron hematoxylin working solution for I minute.
5. Wash in running water for 10 minutes.
6. Rinse in 95% alcohol.
7. Counterstain in methyl orange solution for 5 minutes or until background is light yellow.
8. Dehydrate and clear through 95% ethyl alcohol, absolute ethyl alcohol, and xylene, 2 changes each, 2 minutes each.
9. Mount with resinous medium.

RESULTS

Mast cells .... purple
Elastic fibers .... purple
Other cellular elements .... blue
Background .... yellow

REFERENCE

Luna L. *Manual of Histologic Staining Methods of the Armed Forces Institute of Pathology*. New York, NY: McGraw-Hill; 1968:114-115.

LUNA'S METHOD FOR ERYTHROCYTES & EOSINOPHIL GRANULES

FIXATION: 10% buffered neutral formalin.

SECTIONS: Paraffin, 6 micrometers.

SOLUTIONS
IRON HEMATOXYLIN WORKING SOLUTION, WEIGERT'S (Ch. 3)

1% BIEBRICH SCARLET SOLUTION (Ch. 3)

HEMATOXYLIN-BIEBRICH SCARLET SOLUTION
Weigert's iron hematoxylin working solution ....45.0 ml
Biebrich scarlet solution ....5.0 ml

1% ACID ALCOHOL SOLUTION (Ch. 3)

0.5% LITHIUM CARBONATE SOLUTION (Ch. 3)

PROCEDURE
1. Deparaffinize and hydrate to distilled water.
2. Stain in hematoxylin-Biebrich scarlet solution for 5 minutes.
3. Differentiate in 1% acid alcohol solution to obtain the desired nuclear detail, usually no more than 8 dips.
4. Rinse in tap water.
5. Dip in lithium carbonate solution until sections turn blue and erythrocytes are bright red. Five dips usually suffice.
6. Wash in running water for 2 minutes.
7. Dehydrate and clear through 95% ethyl alcohol, absolute ethyl alcohol and xylene, 2 changes each, 2 minutes each.
8. Mount with resinous medium.

RESULTS
Eosinophil granules	red
Erythrocytes	red
Charcott Leyden crystals	red
Background	blue

REFERENCE
Luna LG. *Manual of histologic staining methods of the Armed Forces Institute of Pathology.* New York, NY: McGraw-Hill; 1968:111.

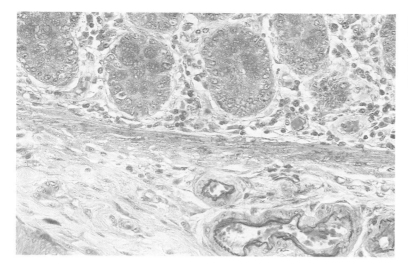

Fig. 17-1.
Movat Stain. Intestine.
Acid mucin, green.
Elastic fibers, black.
Muscle, red brown.
Collagen, yellow.

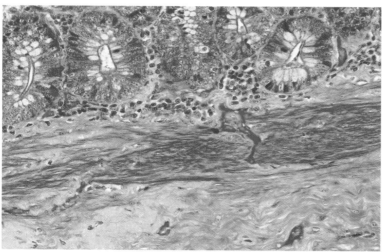

Fig. 17-2.
Masson Stain.
Intestine.
Muscle, red.
Collagen, blue.

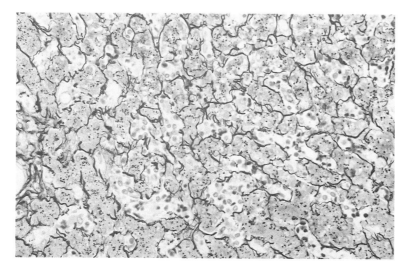

Fig. 17-3.
Manuel's Reticulum
Stain. Liver.

❖ Connective Tissue

CHAPTER 18

CARBOHYDRATES

Elbert Gaffney

A preliminary discussion of carbohydrate complexes as seen in normal body tissues will aid the technologist in the performance and quality control of the special stains which follow. An awareness that these complexes are often altered in disease processes will enhance the performance of those staining procedures which are specific and non specific. Tissues rich in particular carbohydrate complexes are;

GLYCOGEN—Liver, cardiac and skeletal muscle.
SIALOMUCINS—Salivary glands, intestinal goblet cells, gastric lining cells.
NEUTRAL MUCOSUBSTANCE—Gastric lining cells, duodenal Brunner glands.
ACID MUCOSUBSTANCE—Goblet cells of the intestine.
HYALURONIC ACID—Umbilical cord, connective tissue of dermis.
CHONDROITIN SULFATE—Cartilage, aorta, heart valve, umbilical cord, dermis.
HEPARIN SULFATE—Mast cells, aorta, cardiac connective tissue.

Some of the recognized staining procedures for the demonstration of carbohydrate complexes include:

GLYCOGEN, Periodic Acid Schiff (PAS)
NEUTRAL MUCOSUBSTANCES, Periodic Acid Schiff (PAS), with diastase.
ACID MUCOSUBSTANCES, Alcian Blue, pH 2.5 and 0.4
    The different pHs provide differential staining of sulfated (pH 0.4) and non sulfated (pH 2.5) types.
SIALOMUCINS AND SULFATED MUCOSUBSTANCES,
    Gomori's Aldehyde Fuchsin pH 1.7 and pH 1.0.
ACID MUCOSACCHARIDES, Colloidal Iron
CHONDROMUCINS, Safranin O.
HEPARIN SULFATE, Gomori's Aldehyde Fuchsin.

Although a mucicarmine procedure is often requested, we have observed that the results are non-specific for the demonstration of acid mucosubstances. We have also observed that the staining of connective tissue mucosubstances is not as consistent as the staining of epithelial mucosubstances.

The enzymes, diastase, sialidase (neuraminidase), and bovine testicular hyaluronidase will eliminate the staining of glycogen, sialic acid, and hyaluronic acid, respectively. Hyaluronidase will also eliminate staining attributable to Chondroitin Sulfates A and C.

The enzymes pectinase and chondroitinase are not routinely used in our histopathology laboratories. Pectinase will remove all PAS non-glycogen material from tissue sections. Chondroitinase ABC will remove chondroitin sulfates A and C and dermatin sulfate B from tissue sections. Chondroitinase has no effect on hyaluronic acid.

To summarize, diastase (or amylase) removes staining attributed to glycogen;

sialidase (neuraminidase) removes staining attributed to sialomucins; bovine testicular hyaluronidase will remove staining attributed to chondroitin sulfates A & C and hyaluronic acid; and streptococcal and pneumococcal hyaluronidase will remove staining attributed to hyaluronic acid only with no effect on the chondroitin sulfates.

PERIODIC ACID SCHIFF (PAS) PROCEDURE
AFIP Modification of the McManus Procedure

FIXATION: 10% buffered neutral formalin.

SECTIONS: Paraffin, 6 micrometers.

SOLUTIONS
0.5% PERIODIC ACID SOLUTION

Periodic acid ....0.5 gm
Distilled water ....100.0 ml

1N HYDROCHLORIC ACID SOLUTION

Hydrochloric acid, sp. gr. 1.19 ....83.5 ml
Distilled water ....916.5 ml

COLEMAN'S SCHIFF REAGENT

Basic fuchsin ....1.0 gm
Distilled water, heat to 60° ....200.0 ml
Bring just to boiling point.
Cool and then add
Potassium metabisulfite ....2.0 gm
1 N hydrochloric acid ....10.0 ml
Let bleach for 24 hours then add
Carbon, activated ....0.5 gm

Shake for 1 minute, then filter through coarse filter paper. Repeat filtration until solution is colorless. Store in refrigerator.

MAYER'S HEMATOXYLIN SOLUTION (Ch. 9)

OR

HARRIS' HEMATOXYLIN SOLUTION (Ch. 9)

PROCEDURE
1. Deparaffinize and hydrate to water.
2. Oxidize in periodic acid solution for 5 minutes. *10 min.* *lap. ck*
3. Rinse in distilled water.
4. Place in Coleman's Schiff reagent for 15 minutes.
5. Wash in lukewarm tapwater for 10 minutes.
6. Counterstain in Mayer's hematoxylin solution for 15 minutes, or Harris' for 6 minutes. *Gill's ±3 min, wash, blue, wash*
7. Wash in tap water for 15 minutes.
8. Dehydrate and clear through 95% ethyl alcohol, absolute ethyl alcohol, and xylene, 2 changes, 2 minutes each.
9. Mount with resinous medium.

RESULTS   (See Fig. 18-1, page 172).

Glycogen, mucin, and some
 basement membranes ....red to purple
Fungi ....red to purple
Nuclei ....blue

REFERENCE

McManus JFA: Histological and histochemical uses of periodic acid. *Stain Technol.* 1948;23:99.

DIASTASE DIGESTION METHOD

SOLUTIONS

PHOSPHATE BUFFER SOLUTION, pH 6.0

Sodium chloride .... 8.0 gm
Sodium phosphate, dibasic .... 0.28 gm
Sodium phosphate, monobasic .... 1.97 gm
Distilled water .... 100.0 ml

DIASTASE DIGESTION SOLUTION

Diastase of malt .... 0.1 gm
Phosphate buffer solution, pH 6.0 .... 100.0 ml

PROCEDURE
1. Deparaffinize and hydrate to distilled water.
2. Place in preheated, 37°C, diastase digestion solution for 1 hour.
3. Wash thoroughly in running tap water or several changes of distilled water.
4. Proceed with a procedure for glycogen, namely the Periodic Acid Schiff.

RESULTS   (See Figs. 18–1, 2, page 172).
Staining attributed to glycogen is eliminated.

❖ Carbohydrates

MAYER'S MUCICARMINE METHOD

FIXATION: 10% buffered neutral formalin.

SECTIONS: Paraffin, 6 micrometers.

SOLUTIONS

SOUTHGATE'S MUCICARMINE STOCK SOLUTION

Carmine .... 1.0 gm
Aluminum hydroxide .... 1.0 gm
Alcohol, 50% ethyl .... 100.0 ml
Mix in a 500 ml flask. Shake well.
Caution: add small amounts at a time with intermittent shaking.
Aluminum chloride, anhydrous .... 0.5 gm

Preheat a water bath to the boiling point. Place flask in boiling water; bring contents to a rapid boil for 2 to 3 minutes. Cool rapidly under running tap water. When cold, filter and label as Stock, which remains stable for several months.

SOUTHGATE'S MUCICARMINE WORKING SOLUTION

Southgate's mucicarmine stock solution .... 10.0 ml
Distilled water .... 90.0 ml

IRON HEMATOXYLIN (WEIGERT'S) WORKING SOLUTION (Ch.3)

0.25% METANIL YELLOW SOLUTION

Metanil yellow .... 0.25 gm
Distilled water .... 100.0 ml
Acetic acid, glacial .... 0.25 ml

PROCEDURE

1. Deparaffinize and hydrate to water.
2. Weigert's iron hematoxylin working solution for 7 minutes.
3. Rinse briefly in tap water. Then rinse in diluted acid alcohol solution (10 ml of 1% acid alcohol [Ch. 3] and 90 ml distilled water) to clear the background.
4. Wash in running tap water for 10 minutes.
5. Stain in Southgate's mucicarmine working solution for 30 minutes. Discard solution.
6. Rinse quickly in distilled water.
7. Counterstain in metanil yellow solution for 1 minute.
8. Dehydrate and clear through 95% ethyl alcohol, absolute ethyl alcohol, and xylene, 2 changes each, 2 minutes each.
9. Mount with resinous medium.

RESULTS (See Figs. 18–3, 4, page 172).

Mucin ....dark rose

Capsules of cryptococci ....dark rose

Nuclei ....black

Background ....yellow

REFERENCE

Southgate HW: Note on preparing mucicarmine. J Path Bact 1927; 30:729.

ALCIAN BLUE, pH 2.5

FIXATION: 10% buffered neutral formalin.

SECTIONS: Paraffin, 6 micrometers.

SOLUTIONS

3% ACETIC ACID SOLUTION (Ch. 3)

ALCIAN BLUE SOLUTION

Alcian blue, 8GX .... 1.0 gm
Acetic acid, 3% solution .... 100.0 ml

NUCLEAR FAST RED (KERNECHTROT) SOLUTION (Ch. 3)

PROCEDURE
1. Deparaffinize and hydrate to distilled water.
2. Place in 3% acetic acid solution for 3 minutes.
3. Stain in alcian blue solution for 30 minutes.
4. Wash in running water for 10 minutes.
5. Rinse in distilled water.
6. Counterstain in filtered nuclear fast red solution for 5 minutes.
7. Wash in running water for 1 minute.
8. Dehydrate and clear through 95% ethyl alcohol, absolute ethyl alcohol, and xylene, 2 changes each, 2 minutes each.
9. Mount with resinous medium.

RESULTS   (See Fig. 18-5, page 173).
Weakly acidic sulfated mucosubstances,
   hyaluronic acid, and sialomucins .... dark blue
Nuclei .... red to pink
Cytoplasm .... pale pink

REFERENCE
Lev R, Spicer SS. Specific staining of sulfate groups with alcian blue at low pH. *J Histochem Cytochem.* 1964;12:309.

ALCIAN BLUE, pH 1.0

FIXATION: 10% buffered neutral formalin.

SECTIONS: Paraffin, 6 micrometers.

SOLUTIONS

1N HYDROCHLORIC ACID SOLUTION (Ch. 3)

0.1N HYDROCHLORIC ACID SOLUTION

Hydrochloric acid, 1 N ....10.0 ml
Distilled water ....90.0 ml

ALCIAN BLUE SOLUTION

Alcian blue, 8GX ....1.0 gm
Hydrochloric acid, 0.1 N ....100.0 ml

PROCEDURE

1. Deparaffinize and hydrate to distilled water.
2. Stain in alcian blue solution for 30 minutes.
3. Blot sections dry with filter paper without rinsing in water.
4. Dehydrate and clear through 95% ethyl alcohol, absolute ethyl alcohol, and xylene, 2 changes each, 2 minutes each.
5. Mount with resinous medium.

RESULTS

Sulfated mucosubstances ....dark blue

REFERENCE

Lev R, Spicer SS. Specific staining of sulfate groups with alcian blue at low pH. *J Histochem Cytochem.* 1964;12:309.

ALCIAN BLUE, pH 0.4

FIXATION: 10% buffered neutral formalin.

SECTIONS: Paraffin, 6 micrometers.

SOLUTIONS

PHOSPHATE/HYDROCHLORIC ACID SOLUTION

Hydrochloric acid, concentrated ....42.0 ml
Sodium phosphate, monobasic ....13.8 gm
Distilled water ....958.0 ml

ALCIAN BLUE SOLUTION, pH 0.4

Alcian blue, 8GX ....2.5 gm
Phosphate/hydrochloric acid solution ....250.0 ml

NUCLEAR FAST RED (KERNECHTROT) SOLUTION (Ch. 3)

PROCEDURE
1. Deparaffinize and hydrate to distilled water.
2. Phosphate/hydrochloric acid solution for 3 minutes.
3. Stain in alcian blue solution for 30 minutes.
4. Wash in running water for 10 minutes.
5. Rinse in distilled water.
6. Counterstain in nuclear fast red solution for 5 minutes.
7. Wash in running water for 1 minute.
8. Dehydrate and clear through 95% ethyl alcohol, absolute ethyl alcohol, and xylene, 2 changes each, 2 minutes each.
9. Mount with resinous medium.

RESULTS

Strongly acidic sulfated mucosubstances ....blue
Nuclei ....pink to red
Cytoplasm ....pale pink

REFERENCE
Johnson WC, Graham JH, Helwig EB. Histochemistry of the acid mucopolysaccharides in cutaneous calcification. *J Invest Derm*. 1964;42:215.

HYALURONIDASE DIGESTION METHOD

FIXATION: 10% buffered neutral formalin or 95% alcohol.

TECHNIQUE: Paraffin, 6 micrometers.

SOLUTIONS

PHOSPHATE BUFFER SOLUTION

Sodium chloride ....8.0 gm
Sodium phosphate, monobasic ....2.0 gm
Sodium phosphate, dibasic......................................0.3 gm
Distilled water ....1000.0 ml

HYALURONIDASE DIGESTION SOLUTION

Hyaluronidase, bovine testicular ....0.05 gm
Buffer solution ....100.0 ml

PROCEDURE

1. Deparaffinize and hydrate 2 serial sections to distilled water.
2. Incubate 1 section in the hyaluronidase solution at 37°C for 1 hour and the duplicate section in phosphate buffer solution at 37°C for 1 hour.
3. Wash both slides in running water for 5 minutes.
4. Stain as desired.

RESULTS   (See Figs. 18–5, 6, page 173).
Staining attributable to hyaluronic acid, chondroitin-4-sulfate or chondroitin-6-sulfate is eliminated by hyaluronidase digestion.

ALCIAN BLUE – PAS, pH 2.5 or pH 1.0

FIXATION: 10% buffered neutral formalin.

SECTIONS: Paraffin, 4-6 micrometers.

SOLUTIONS

ALCIAN BLUE 8GX SOLUTION, pH 2.5 or 1.0
(see Alcian blue procedures , above)

1% PERIODIC ACID SOLUTION

Periodic acid ....1.0 gm
Distilled water ....100.0 ml

COLEMAN'S SCHIFF REAGENT (see PAS procedure, above)

PROCEDURE
1. Deparaffinize and hydrate slides to distilled water.
2. Stain in alcian blue 8GX solution (pH 2.5 or pH 1.0) for 30 minutes.
3. Wash alcian blue 8GX, pH 2.5 sections in tap water for 5 minutes **or** blot the alcian blue 8GX, pH 1.0 sections until dry.
4. Place in periodic acid solution for 10 minutes.
5. Wash in tap water for 5 minutes.
6. Place in Coleman's Schiff reagent solution for 10 minutes.
7. Wash in lukewarm tap water for 10 minutes.
8. Dehydrate and clear through 95% ethyl alcohol, absolute ethyl alcohol, and xylene, two changes each, 2 minutes each.
9. Mount using resinous medium.

RESULTS
AB(pH 2.5) - PAS: hyaluronic acid and sialomucins ....blue
AB(pH 1.0) - PAS: sulfated mucosubstances ....blue
Polysaccharides and neutral mucosubstances
containing hexoses and deoxyhexoses with
vicinal glycol groups ....magenta to red

REFERENCE
Lev R, Spicer SS. Specific staining of sulfate groups with alcian blue at low pH. *J Histochem Cytochem.* 1964;12:309.

SIALIDASE DIGESTION METHOD

SOLUTIONS

BUFFER SOLUTION A

Sodium acetate .... 26.2 gm
Calcium chloride .... 8.9 gm
Distilled water .... 200.0 ml

BUFFER SOLUTION B

Sodium acetate .... 26.0 gm
Calcium chloride .... 0.8 gm
Distilled water .... 200.0 ml

SIALIDASE (NEURAMINIDASE) DIGESTION SOLUTION

Sialidase (Neuraminidase) .... 1.0 ml
Buffer solution A .... 0.1 ml

PROCEDURE
1. Deparaffinize and hydrate to distilled water two slides; one to be digested and the other undigested.
2. Circle the entire section, on both slides, with a diamond marking pen.
3. Air dry slides for at least 2 hours.[a]
4. Place slides on glass rods in a dish which can be covered.[b]
5. Cover the slide marked for digestion with the sialidase digestion solution. Cover the undigested slide with buffer solution B.
6. Both slides should be left covered for 3 hours at room temperature.[c]
7. Rinse with distilled water.
8. Perform any of the requested mucopolysaccharide staining procedures.

RESULTS

Staining attributed to sialomucins will be eliminated.

[a]It may be advantageous to take slides through step 3 and then leave overnight. The following morning start at step 4.

[b]To prevent the drying of the sialidase digestion solution, insert moist paper towels in the bottom of the dish, then put the glass rods in place.

[c]The sections must be covered to prevent the drying of the digestion solution.

MOWRY'S COLLOIDAL IRON

FIXATION: 10% buffered neutral formalin. Bichromate fixatives should be avoided.

SECTIONS: Paraffin, 6 micrometers.

SOLUTIONS

29% FERRIC CHLORIDE SOLUTION (Ch. 3)

MÜLLER'S COLLOIDAL IRON STOCK SOLUTION

Distilled water .... 250.0 ml
Bring to a boil. Add:
Ferric chloride solution, 29% .... 4.4 ml

MÜLLER'S COLLOIDAL IRON WORKING SOLUTION

Müller's colloidal iron, stock .... 20.0 ml
Distilled water .... 15.0 ml
Acetic acid, glacial .... 5.0 ml

12% ACETIC ACID SOLUTION (Ch. 3)

5% POTASSIUM FERROCYANIDE STOCK SOLUTION (Ch. 3)

5 % HYDROCHLORIC ACID STOCK SOLUTION (Ch. 3)

POTASSIUM FERROCYANIDE/HYDROCHLORIC ACID WORKING SOLUTION

Potassium ferrocyanide, 5% stock .... 40.0 ml
Hydrochloric acid, 5% stock .... 40.0 ml

VAN GIESON SOLUTION (Ch. 3)

OR

NUCLEAR FAST RED SOLUTION (Ch. 3)

PROCEDURE
1. Deparaffinize and hydrate to distilled water.
2. 12% acetic acid solution for 3 minutes.
3. Stain in Müller's colloidal iron working solution for 1 hour.
4. Rinse in 12% acetic acid solution, 4 changes, for 3 minutes each.
5. Potassium ferrocyanide/hydrochloric acid working solution for 20 minutes.
6. Wash in tap water for 5 minutes.
7. Rinse in distilled water.
8. Counterstain in van Gieson solution for 5-7 minutes, or nuclear fast red solution for 5 minutes, which shows greater tissue detail.

9. Dehydrate and clear through 95% ethyl alcohol, absolute ethyl alcohol, and xylene, 2 changes each, for 2 minutes each.
10. Mount with resinous medium.

RESULTS   (See Fig. 18–7, page 173).
Acidic mucopolysaccharides ....blue

REFERENCE
McManus JFA, Mowry RW. *Staining Methods Histologic and Histochemical.* New York, NY: Hoeber; 1960:133.

COLLOIDAL IRON–PAS

FIXATION: 10% buffered neutral formalin.

SECTIONS: Paraffin, 4 to 6 micrometers.

SOLUTIONS

29% FERRIC CHLORIDE SOLUTION (Ch. 3)

MÜLLER'S COLLOIDAL IRON STOCK SOLUTION

Distilled water .... 250.0 ml
Bring to a boil. Add:
Ferric chloride solution, 29% .... 4.4 ml

MÜLLER'S COLLOIDAL IRON WORKING SOLUTION

Müller's colloidal iron, stock .... 20.0 ml
Distilled water .... 15.0 ml
Acetic acid, glacial .... 5.0 ml

12% ACETIC ACID SOLUTION (Ch. 3)

POTASSIUM FERROCYANIDE/HYDROCHLORIC ACID WORKING SOLUTION (see Mowry's colloidal iron procedure above)

0.5% PERIODIC ACID SOLUTION (Ch. 3)

COLEMAN'S SCHIFF REAGENT

Basic fuchsin .... 1.0 gm
Distilled water, heat to 60° .... 200.0 ml
Bring just to boiling point.
Cool and then add
Potassium metabisulfite .... 2.0 gm
1 N hydrochloric acid .... 10.0 ml
Let bleach for 24 hours then add
Carbon, activated .... 0.5 gm

Shake for 1 minute, then filter through coarse filter paper. Repeat filtration until solution is colorless. Store in refrigerator.

PROCEDURE
1. Deparaffinize and hydrate to distilled water.
2. Place in 12% acetic acid solution for 3 minutes.
3. Stain in Müller's colloidal iron working solution for 1 hour.
4. Rinse in 4 changes of 12% acetic acid solution, 3 minutes each.

5. Place in potassium ferrocyanide/hydrochloric acid working solution for 20 minutes.
6. Wash in running tap water for 5 minutes then place in distilled water.
7. Oxidize in periodic acid solution for 5 minutes.
8. Rinse in 3 changes of distilled water.
9. Place in Coleman's Schiff reagent for 10 minutes.
10. Wash in lukewarm running tap water for 5 minutes.
11. Rinse in distilled water.
12. Dehydrate and clear through 95% ethyl alcohol, absolute ethyl alcohol, and xylene, 2 changes each, 2 minutes each.
13. Mount using resinous medium.

RESULTS   (See Fig. 18–8, page 173).

Acid mucosubstances ....deep blue
Neutral mucosubstances,
    containing hexoses ....red to magenta

---

REFERENCES

Mowry RW. Improved procedure for the staining of acidic polysaccharides by Müller's colloidal (hydrous) ferric oxide and its combination with the feulgen and the periodic acid-schiff reaction. *Lab Invest.* 1958;7:566.

McManus JFA. Histological and histochemical uses of periodic acid. *Stain Technol.* 1948;23:99.

ALDEHYDE FUCHSIN, pH 1.0

FIXATION: 10% buffered neutral formalin.

TECHNIQUE: Paraffin, 6 micrometers.

SOLUTIONS
ALDEHYDE FUCHSIN SOLUTION

Basic fuchsin .... 1.0 gm
Alcohol, 70% .... 200.0 ml
Hydrochloric acid, concentrated .... 2.0 ml
Paraldehyde .... 2.0 ml

Let stand at room temperature for 2 to 5 days until stain is deep purple. This solution has a pH of 1.7. To adjust the pH to 1.0, use concentrated hydrochloric acid. A properly made solution will form a metallic sheen on the sides of bottle.

0.25% METANIL YELLOW SOLUTION

Metanil yellow .... 0.25 gm
Deionized water .... 100.0 ml
Acetic acid, glacial .... 0.25 ml

1% ACID ALCOHOL

Alcohol, 70% .... 99.0 ml
Hydrochloric acid, concentrated .... 1.0 ml

NUCLEAR FAST RED SOLUTION (Ch. 3)

PROCEDURE
1. Deparaffinize sections and hydrate to deionized water.
2. Rinse in three changes of acid alcohol solution.
3. Stain in aldehyde fuchsin solution (pH 1.0) for 30 minutes.
4. Rinse off excess stain in acid alcohol solution.
5. Counterstain with metanil yellow solution for 1 minute or until background is a pale yellow.
6. Rinse in 2 changes of deionized water.
7. Stain in nuclear fast red solution for 1-3 minutes to stain nuclei.
8. Rinse in 2 changes of deionized water.
9. Dehydrate in 2 changes each of 95% alcohol and absolute ethyl alcohol, and clear in 2 changes of xylene.
10. Mount with resinous mounting media.

RESULTS   (See Fig. 18–9, page 174).
Highly acidic sulfated mucosubstances .... purple

REFERENCE
Johnson WC, Graham JH, and Helwig EB. Histochemistry of the acid mucopolysaccharides in cutaneous calcification. *J Invest Derm.* 1964;42:215.

SAFRANIN O METHOD

FIXATION: 10% buffered neutral formalin.

SECTIONS: Paraffin, 6 micrometers.

SOLUTIONS

IRON HEMATOXYLIN (WEIGERT'S) WORKING SOLUTION (Ch. 3)

0.001% FAST GREEN (FCF) SOLUTION

Fast green, FCF, C.I. 42053 .... 0.1 gm
Distilled water .... 1000.0 ml

1% ACETIC ACID SOLUTION

Acetic acid, glacial .... 1.0 ml
Distilled water .... 99.0 ml

0.1% SAFRANIN O SOLUTION

Safranin 0, C.I. 50240 .... 0.1 gm
Distilled water .... 100.0 ml

PROCEDURE

1. Deparaffinize and hydrate to water.
2. Stain with Weigert's iron hematoxylin working solution for 7 minutes.
3. Wash in running tap water for 10 minutes.
4. Stain with fast green (FCF) solution for 3 minutes.
5. Rinse quickly with 1% acetic acid solution for no more than 10 to 15 seconds.
6. Stain in 0.1% safranin O solution for 5 minutes.
7. Dehydrate and clear with 95% ethyl alcohol, absolute ethyl alcohol, and xylene, using 2 changes each, 2 minutes each.
8. Mount using resinous medium.

RESULTS   (See Fig. 18–10, page 174).

Nuclei .... black
Cytoplasm .... gray green
Cartilage, mucin, mast cell granules .... orange to red

---

REFERENCES

Lillie RD, Fulmer HM. *Histopathologic Technic and Practical Histochemistry*, 4th ed. New York, NY: McGraw-Hill; 1976:657.

Conn HJ, Lillie RD. *Biological Stains*, 9th ed. Baltimore, Md: Waverly Press; 1977:387.

CONGO RED (BENNHOLD'S) METHOD FOR AMYLOID

FIXATION: 10% buffered neutral formalin.

SECTIONS: Paraffin, 6 to 12[a] micrometers.

SOLUTIONS

1% CONGO RED SOLUTION

Congo red .... 1.0 gm
Distilled water .... 100.0 ml

1% SODIUM HYDROXIDE SOLUTION

Sodium hydroxide .... 1.0 gm
Distilled water .... 100.0 ml

ALKALINE ALCOHOL SOLUTION

Sodium hydroxide solution, 1% .... 1.0 ml
Ethyl alcohol solution, 50% .... 99.0 ml

MAYER'S HEMATOXYLIN SOLUTION (Ch. 9)

PROCEDURE
1. Deparaffinize and hydrate to distilled water.
2. Stain in filtered Congo red solution for 1 hour.
3. Rinse briefly in distilled water.
4. Differentiate rapidly in alkaline alcohol solution.
5. Wash in running tap water for 5 minutes.
6. Counterstain in Mayer's hematoxylin solution for 5 minutes. *Gill's - 1 min.*
7. Wash in running tap water for 15 minutes. *8 min to blue slides*
8. Dehydrate and clear through 95% ethyl, absolute ethyl alcohol, and xylene, 2 changes each, 2 minutes each. *reg. dehydration routine*
9. Mount using resinous medium.

RESULTS   (See Fig. 18-11, 12, page 174).
Amyloid .... pink to red, and "apple-green"
birefringence with polarized light
Nuclei .... blue

[a]In cases of suspected amyloidosis, thick sections at 12 micrometers may be beneficial in demonstrating minute deposits of amyloid.

CRYSTAL VIOLET (LIEB'S) METHOD FOR AMYLOID

FIXATION: 10% buffered neutral formalin.

SECTIONS: Paraffin, 4 to 6 micrometers.

SOLUTIONS

CRYSTAL VIOLET STOCK SOLUTION

Crystal violet .... 14.0 gm
Alcohol, 95% ethyl .... 100.0 ml

CRYSTAL VIOLET WORKING SOLUTION

Crystal violet solution, stock .... 10.0 ml
Distilled water .... 300.0 ml
Hydrochloric acid, concentrated .... 1.0 ml

APATHY'S MOUNTING MEDIUM (Ch. 10)

PROCEDURE

1. Deparaffinize and hydrate to distilled water.
2. Stain in crystal violet working solution for 5 hours.
3. Wash in running tap water for 15 minutes.
4. Mount with aqueous mounting medium such as, Apathy's, or sections may be air dried for 15 minutes or longer, dipped in xylene and coverslipped with a resinous medium.
5. Examine without delay as stain may fade.

RESULTS

Amyloid .... purple violet
Other tissue elements .... blue

REFERENCES

Lieb E. Permanent stain for amyloid. *Amer J Clin Pathol.* 1947;17:413.

Sheehan DC, Hrapchak BB. *Theory and Practice of Histotechnology*, 2nd ed. Columbus, Ohio: Battelle Press; 1980:176-177.

SIRIUS RED METHOD FOR AMYLOID

FIXATION: 10% buffered neutral formalin.

SECTIONS: Paraffin, 4-6 micrometers.

SOLUTIONS

1% SODIUM HYDROXIDE SOLUTION

Sodium hydroxide .... 1.0 gm
Distilled water .... 100.0 ml

ALKALINE ALCOHOL SOLUTION

Alcohol, 80% ethyl .... 100.0 ml
Sodium hydroxide, 1% .... 1.0 ml

SIRIUS RED SOLUTION

Sirius Red, F3BA .... 1.0 gm
Distilled water .... 100.0 ml
Dissolve and then add:
Sodium chloride .... 0.5 gm
Let stand overnight before use. DO NOT FILTER.

0.1 M BORATE BUFFER SOLUTION, pH 9.0

Sodium borate .... 38.1 gm
Distilled water .... 1000.0 ml

MAYER'S HEMATOXYLIN SOLUTION (Ch. 9)

PROCEDURE
1. Deparaffinize and hydrate slides to distilled water.
2. Wash in running tap water for 5 minutes.
3. Place in buffered neutral formalin solution overnight.
4. Wash in tap water for 15 minutes.
5. Place in alkaline alcohol solution for 1 hour.
6. Rinse quickly in distilled water for 10 seconds.
7. Place in preheated (60°C) sirius red solution in a 60°C oven for 90 minutes.
8. Rinse quickly in two changes of the borate buffer solution.
9. Wash in running water for 5 minutes.
10. Stain in Mayer's hematoxylin solution for 5 minutes.
11. Wash in running tap water for 15 minutes.
12. Drain slides and dehydrate and clear rapidly through two changes each of absolute ethyl alcohol and xylene.
13. Mount using resinous medium.

RESULTS

Amyloid and elastin .... pink to red
Nuclei .... blue
Background .... unstained
Cellulose, including cotton fibers .... pink to red

REFERENCE

Sweat F, Puchtler H. Demonstration of amyloid with direct cotton dyes. *Arch Path.* 1965;80:613.

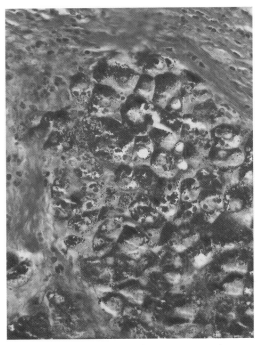

Fig. 18-1. PAS preparation. Large amount of glycogen in liver cells.

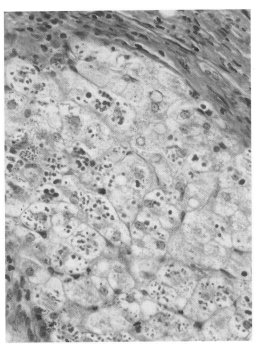

Fig. 18-2. PAS preparation after diastase treatment of section adjacent to that in 18-1. Glycogen has been removed. PAS-positive globules remain, characteristic of alpha-1-antitrypsin deficiency.

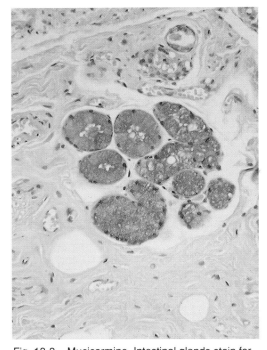

Fig. 18-3. Mucicarmine. Intestinal glands stain for mucin.

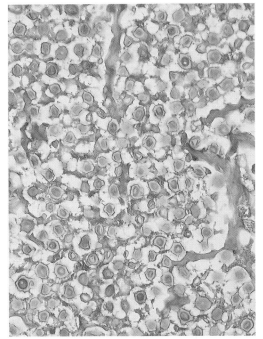

Fig. 18-4. Mucicarmine. Capsules of cryptococci stain red.

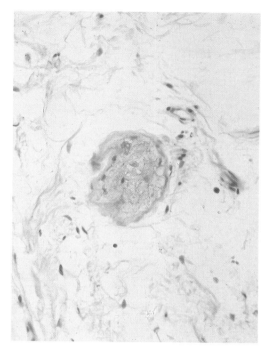

Fig. 18-5.   Alcian blue, pH 2.5. Nerve with connective tissue mucin.

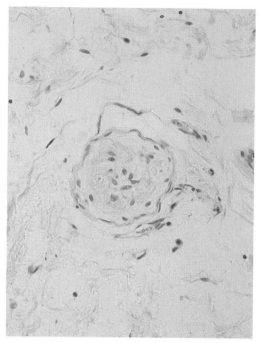

Fig. 18-6.   Alcian blue, pH 2.5 after I hour digestion with hyaluronidase. Mucin is diminished compared to Fig. 18-5.

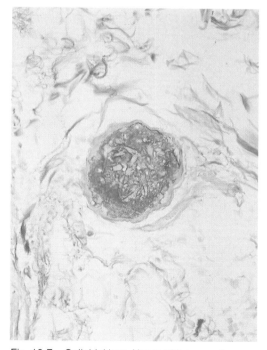

Fig. 18-7.   Colloidal iron. Nerve with connective tissue mucin.

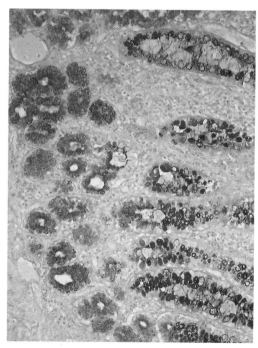

Fig. 18-8.   Colloidal iron-PAS. Intestinal glands with neutral (red) and acid (blue) mucin.

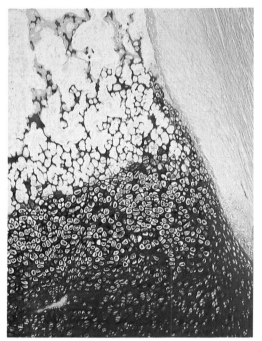

Fig.18-9. Aldehyde fuchsin, pH1.0. Developing fetal bone stains for chondromucin.

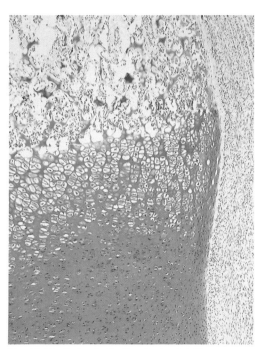

Fig. 18-10. Safranin O. Developing fetal bone stains for chondromucin.

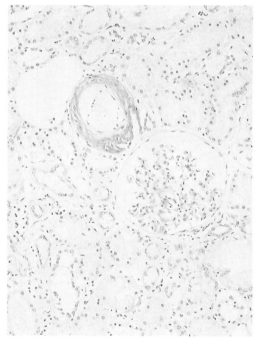

Fig.18-11. Congo red stains amyloid in blood vessels and glomerulus.

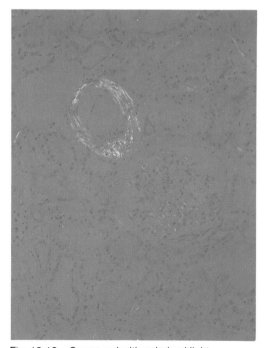

Fig. 18-12. Congo red with polarized light shows "apple-green" birefringence of amyloid.

❖ CHAPTER 19

LIPIDS

Frank B. Johnson

Lipids are substances that are insoluble in water but soluble in "fat solvents" such as ethyl alcohol, the xylenes, chloroform, benzene, and gasoline. Lipid stains are usually performed on frozen sections of tissues fixed in buffered neutral formalin. Phospholipids are better preserved in formol calcium; they tend to be leached out by prolonged exposure to buffered neutral formalin. Lipids may be classified as follows, according to a scheme modified from Cain.

CLASSIFICATION	HELPFUL TECHNIQUES AND REACTIONS
A. Paraffins (petrolatum and motor oil)	A. Stainable with oil red O but not with OsO_4
B. Isoprene derivatives (related to vitamin A and the retinoids)	B. Fleeting fluorescence
C. Fatty acids and their derivatives: 1. Fatty acids - saturated or unsaturated 2. Triglycerides - neutral fats (fatty acids joined with glycerol) 3. Waxes - fatty acids joined with long-chained alcohols 4. Phospholipids - fatty acids joined with substances containing phosphoric groups and possible sugars, amino acids, and rarely, sulfate groups	C. Fatty acids and their derivatives generally stain with oil red O and OsO_4 Phospholipids tend to bind metal ions such as chromium and copper. They stain in the Baker acid hematin procedure and with Luxol fast blue (see Ch. 14). The phospholipid of Gaucher disease contains a sugar and is PAS-positive.
D. Lipid peroxides - oxidation products of unsaturated fatty acids or their derivatives	D. May appear to be PAS-positive, but may stain with Schiff reagent without treatment with periodic acid.

| E. Cholesterol and its esters | E. Positive with Schultz reaction |
| F. Lipogenous pigments - not clearly defined chemically. Mixtures or oxidation and polymerization products of unsaturated fatty acids and their derivatives, including ceroid and lipofuscin. | F. May be present in paraffin sections. See chapter on pigments for procedures. |

REFERENCE

Cain AJ. The histochemistry of lipoids in animals. *Biol Rev Cambr Philos Soc.* 1950;25:73.

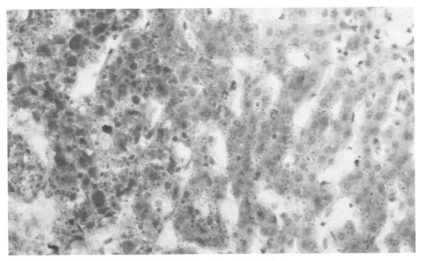

Fig. 19-1. Oil red O. Liver, frozen section. Positive for fat.

AFIP Laboratory Methods in Histotechnology

OIL RED O METHOD FOR FROZEN SECTIONS

FIXATION: 10% buffered neutral formalin.

SECTIONS: Frozen, 4 to 6 micrometers.

SOLUTIONS

100% PROPYLENE GLYCOL

0.5% OIL RED O SOLUTION

Oil red O .... 0.5 gm
Propylene glycol, 100% .... 100.0 ml

Add a small amount to propylene glycol to the oil red O and mix well, crush larger pieces. Gradually add the remainder of the propylene glycol stirring periodically. Heat gently until the solution reaches 95°C. Do not allow to go over 100°C. Stir while heating. Pass through coarse filter paper while still warm. Allow to stand overnight at room temperature. Filter through medium fritted glass filter with the aid of vacuum. If solution becomes turbid, refilter.

85% PROPYLENE GLYCOL SOLUTION

Propylene glycol, 100% .... 85.0 ml
Distilled water .... 15.0 ml

MAYER'S HEMATOXYLIN SOLUTION (see Ch. 9)

GLYCERIN JELLY

Gelatin .... 10.0 gm
Distilled water .... 60.0 ml
Heat until the gelatin is dissolved, then add:
Glycerin .... 70.0 ml
Phenol .... 1.0 ml

PROCEDURE
1. Rinse the slides containing the frozen sections in distilled water.
2. Place in absolute propylene glycol for 2 minutes.
3. Stain in oil red O solution for 16 hours.
4. Differentiate in 85% propylene glycol solution for 1 minute.
5. Rinse in 2 changes of distilled water.
6. Stain in Mayer's hematoxylin solution for 15 to 60 seconds.
7. Rinse thoroughly in several changes of distilled water.
8. Mount in warmed glycerin jelly solution.

RESULTS   (See Fig. 19–1, page 176).

Lipids .... red
Nuclei .... blue

❖ Lipids

OIL RED O FOR PARAFFIN SECTIONS

FIXATION: 10% buffered neutral formalin.

SECTIONS: Paraffin, 4 to 10 micrometers.

SOLUTIONS

100% PROPYLENE GLYCOL

0.5% OIL RED O SOLUTION

Oil red O ....0.5 gm
Propylene glycol, 100% ....100.0 ml

Add a small amount to propylene glycol to the oil red O and mix well, crush larger pieces. Gradually add the remainder of the propylene glycol stirring periodically. Heat gently until the solution reaches 95°C. Do not allow to go over 100°C. Stir while heating. Pass through coarse filter paper while still warm. Allow to stand overnight at room temperature. Filter through medium fritted glass filter with the aid of vacuum. If solution becomes turbid, refilter.

85% PROPYLENE GLYCOL SOLUTION

Propylene glycol, 100% ....85.0 ml
Distilled water ....15.0 ml

MAYER'S HEMATOXYLIN SOLUTION (see Ch. 9)

GLYCERIN JELLY

Gelatin ....10.0 gm
Distilled water ....60.0 ml
Heat until the gelatin is dissolved, then add:
Glycerin ....70.0 ml
Phenol ....1.0 ml

PROCEDURE
1. Deparaffinize and hydrate to distilled water.
2. Place in absolute propylene glycol for 3 to 5 minutes.
3. Stain in oil red O solution for 48 to 72 hours.
4. Rinse in 85% propylene glycol solution for 1 to 2 minutes.
5. Stain in Mayer's hematoxylin solution for 5 minutes.
6. Wash thoroughly in running water for 3 minutes.
7. Rinse in 2 changes of distilled water.
8. Mount with glycerin jelly.

RESULTS
Lipids...red
Nuclei...pale blue

OSMIUM TETROXIDE METHOD FOR FAT IN FROZEN SECTIONS

FIXATION: 10% buffered neutral formalin.

SECTIONS: Frozen, 4 to 6 micrometers.

SOLUTIONS

1% OSMIUM TETROXIDE

Osmium tetroxide, ampule .... 1.0 gm
Distilled water .... 100.0 ml

Score a 1-gm ampule of osmium tetroxide with a file and, working under a hood, drop the ampule into a container of distilled water and close it.
USE EXTREME CAUTION. DO NOT INHALE VAPORS.

GLYCERIN JELLY

Gelatin .... 10.0 gm
Distilled water .... 60.0 ml
Heat until the gelatin is dissolved, then add:
Glycerin .... 70.0 ml
Phenol .... 1.0 ml

PROCEDURE

1. Place sections in the 1% osmium tetroxide solution in a closed container under a hood for 24 hours.
2. Wash very thoroughly in several changes of water for 6 hours.
3. Counterstaining is optional.[a]
4. Rinse in distilled water.
5. Mount with glycerin jelly.

RESULTS

Lipids .... black

[a]Optional counterstains include eosin for general background staining or nuclear fast red for nuclear staining.

BAKER ACID HEMATIN FOR PHOSPHOLIPIDS

FIXATION: Formol calcium solution.

SECTIONS: Frozen at 6 to 12 micrometers.

SOLUTIONS

FORMOL-CALCIUM SOLUTION

Formaldehyde 37% ....10.0 ml
Calcium chloride, anhydrous ....10.0 ml
Distilled water ....80.0 ml

DICHROMATE SOLUTION

Potassium dichromate..5.0 gm
Calcium chloride...1.0 gm
Distilled water ....100.0 ml

GELATIN EMBEDDING MEDIUM

Dissolve 25 gm gelatin in 100 ml of distilled water at 60°C with stirring.

ACID HEMATIN SOLUTION

Hematoxylin ....0.1 gm
Distilled water ....98.0 ml
Sodium iodate, 1% ....2.0 ml
Heat to boiling then cool and add:
Glacial acetic acid ....2.0 ml

BORAX FERRICYANIDE SOLUTION

Potassium ferricyanide ....2.5 gm
Sodium borate, tetradecahydrate, crystals ....2.5 gm
Distilled water ....100.0 ml

PROCEDURE

1. Fix fresh tissue blocks in formol-calcium solution for 6 hours.
2. Transfer tissue without washing into dichromate solution for 18 hours
3. Transfer tissue into fresh dichromate solution for 24 hours at 60°C.
4. Wash tissue in tap water for 6 hours.
5. Infiltrate tissue with gelatin embedding medium overnight at 37°C.
6. Remove gelatin block from the incubator and harden in the refrigerator at 4°C. Trim tissue blocks and harden in formol-calcium solution at room temperature. Tissue blocks should remain in formol-calcium solution about 24 hours before cutting; however, they can be left longer in the solution.
7. Wash tissue blocks in tap water for 30 minutes.
8. Cut frozen section at 6-12 micrometers.
9. Place sections in dichromate solution for 1 hour at 60°C.
10. Wash 5 minutes in running tap water; rinse in distilled water.
11. Stain sections in acid hematin solution overnight at 37°C.

AFIP Laboratory Methods in Histotechnology

12. Rinse sections in 2 changes of distilled water and differentiate in borax ferricyanide solution for 30 minutes to 1 hour at 37°C.
13. Wash in running tap water for 5 minutes; rinse in 3 changes of distilled water.
14. Float sections on slide, drain for short time and mount in aqueous medium.

RESULTS

Phospholipids ....blue-black
Background ....brown

Buffered neutral formalin tends to leach phospholipids from tissues. Formol-calcium even when used after initial buffered neutral formalin can give good preservation of phospholipids. Phospholipids can sometimes be demonstrated in paraffin sections of buffered neutral formalin fixed sections. The hydrated sections of such tissue can be carried through steps 1 to 4, then steps 9-13, followed by mounting in aqueous medium.

REFERENCE
Baker JR. The histochemical recognition of lipids. *Quart J Micr Sci.* 1946;87:409.

SCHULTZ METHOD FOR CHOLESTEROL

FIXATION: 10% buffered neutral formalin.

SECTIONS: Frozen, 6 to 10 micrometers.

SOLUTIONS

2.5% FERRIC AMMONIUM SULFATE SOLUTION

Ferric ammonium sulfate ....2.5 gm
Distilled water ....100.0 ml

GLACIAL ACETIC-SULFURIC ACID SOLUTION

Acetic acid, glacial ....50.0 ml
Sulfuric acid, concentrated ....50.0 ml

Place the acetic acid in a beaker that is cooled with ice. Slowly add the concentrated sulfuric acid to the acetic acid, stirring constantly. Prepare just before using.

PROCEDURE

1. Cut frozen sections and collect in distilled water.
2. Mount individual sections onto clean glass slides.
3. Drain and blot dry.
4. Place the slides in the 2.5% ferric ammonium sulfate solution; allow them to remain in the ferric ammonium sulfate solution for 3 days.
5. Rinse in 3 changes of distilled water.
6. Drain and air-dry.
7. Place one drop of the freshly prepared glacial acetic-sulfuric acid solution onto the section.
8. Coverslip the section immediately.
9. Examine microscopically within several minutes.

RESULTS

Cholesterol ....blue to green
Background ....clear

REFERENCES

Schultz A. Eine methode des mikrochemischen cholestrinnachweises am gewebsschnitt. *Zentrabl Allg Pathol.* 1924;35:314.

Reiner CB. The histochemical reaction for cholesterol. *Lab Invest.* 1953;2:140.

❖ CHAPTER 20

PIGMENTS AND MINERALS

Frank B. Johnson

Pigments are substances that have inherent color. The most commonly encountered pigments in pathologic tissues are brown or black. An important differentiation that must be made is between **melanin**, a product of oxidation and polymerization of the amino acid tyrosine and **lipofuscin**, a product of oxidation and polymerization of unsaturated lipids. Both pigments are non-birefringent, brown to black, and iron negative. The following table can help to distinguish these two:

PROCEDURE	MELANIN	LIPOFUSCIN (Ceroid)
PAS	-	-/+
Oil red O	-	-/+
Ammoniacal silver reduction	+	-/+
Acid fast	-	-/+

Lipofuscin is a family of substances of varying composition. Most regard ceroid to be a member of this family. It is usually possible to rule out melanin by observing the positive results with two or more of the above methods. The so-called melanin bleaches may also bleach lipofuscin. The silver reduction method (Warthin-Starry at pH 3.2) was designed to have some specificity for melanin.

The yellow pigments bilirubin and hematoidin are break-down products of hemoglobin and chemically are essentially identical. Sometimes hematoidin is birefringent. Frequently, these pigments can be identified by the stable Gmelin reaction.

Methods for minerals in tissues have not received the attention which they deserve. Many inorganic compounds of interest are highly water soluble, cannot be localized in buffered formalin-fixed tissues, and cannot be stained in aqueous media. Other inorganic compounds are highly water insoluble but unreactive to reagents compatible with tissue preservation. Silica is an example. Some compounds such as the mineral apatite (the inorganic constituent of bone, teeth, and pathologic calcifications) are fairly insoluble but also reactive to non-destructive staining procedures. Some inorganic elements are bound to protein or other organic molecules, which are preserved in formalin-fixed tissues. Some of these can be localized and suitably stained. The x-ray analytic techniques of scanning electron microscopy are tending to inhibit further development of histochemical methods for minerals, but they provide for tests of specificity of methods.

WARTHIN-STARRY METHOD (pH 3.2) FOR MELANIN
AFIP Modification

FIXATION: 10% buffered neutral formalin. Avoid chromate fixatives.

SECTIONS: Paraffin, 4 to 6 micrometers.

SOLUTIONS

1% CITRIC ACID SOLUTION

Citric acid ....1.0 gm
Distilled water ....100.0 ml

WATER FOR INJECTION, USP

ACIDULATED WATER SOLUTION

Water for Injection, USP ....1000.0 ml
Add enough 1% citric acid solution to bring pH to 3.2.

1% SILVER NITRATE SOLUTION (FOR IMPREGNATION)

Silver nitrate, ACS crystals...1.0 gm
Acidulated water solution ....100.0 ml

Preheat a water bath to 43°C. Place a Coplin jar filled with this 1% silver nitrate solution into the water bath. See step 3 of procedure.

2% SILVER NITRATE STOCK SOLUTION (FOR DEVELOPING)

Silver nitrate, ACS crystals...2.0 gm
Acidulated water ....100.0 ml

Prepare fresh. Label a Coplin jar containing this solution. Place in a water bath heated to 54°C. Heat for 30 minutes before using.

5% GELATIN STOCK SOLUTION (FOR DEVELOPING)

Gelatin, 275 Bloom, Type A ....5.0 gm
Acidulated water ....100.0 ml

Prepare fresh. Label a Coplin jar containing this solution. Place in the 54°C water bath and heat solution as indicated above.

0.15% HYDROQUINONE STOCK SOLUTION (FOR DEVELOPING)

Hydroquinone crystals, photographic grade ....0.15 gm
Acidulated water ....100.0 ml

Prepare fresh. Label a Coplin jar containing this solution. Place in the 54°C water bath and heat solution as indicated above.

AFIP Laboratory Methods in Histotechnology

WORKING DEVELOPING SOLUTION

Silver nitrate, 2% stock solution, heated ....1.5 ml
Gelatin, 5% stock solution, heated ....3.75 ml
Hydroquinone, 0.15 stock solution, heated ....2.0 ml

Using a pipette, combine the above, in the order given, in a small flask or beaker approximately 3 to 5 minutes before the end of step 3 of the procedure which follows. Thoroughly mix the silver and gelatin solutions before adding the hydroquinone solution. Then mix all three solutions thoroughly.

NUCLEAR FAST RED SOLUTION (Ch. 3)

PROCEDURE
1. Deparaffinize and hydrate slides to distilled water.
2. Place slides in Water for Injection (USP).
3. Impregnate with 1% silver nitrate solution, at 43°C, for 45 minutes. Prepare the working developing solution 3 to 5 minutes before the end of step 3.
4. Quick-rinse slides, one at a time, in distilled water.
5. Flood slides, which have been placed on a glass rod rack, with the developing solution. Develop for approximately 8 minutes.
6. Wash quickly and thoroughly in hot tap water.
7. Collect all slides in distilled water.
8. Counterstain with nuclear fast red solution for 5 minutes.
9. Rinse in 3 changes of distilled water.
10. Dehydrate and clear through 95% ethyl alcohol, absolute ethyl alcohol, and xylene, 2 changes each, for 2 minutes each.
11. Mount with resinous medium.
12. Discard all solutions used in the preparation of the developing solution.

RESULTS   (See Fig. 20–1, page 200).

Melanin ....black
Nuclei...pink
Cytoplasm ....yellow

REFERENCES

Bridges CH, Luna LG. Kerr's improved Warthin-Starry technic: a study of permissible variations. *Lab Invest.* 1957;6:357.

Faulkner RR, Lillie RD. A buffer modification of the Warthin-Starry method for spirochetes in single paraffin sections. *Stain Technol.* 1945;20:81.

Warkel RL, Luna LG, Helwig EB. A modified Warthin-Starry procedure at low pH for melanin. *Am J Clin Pathol.* 1980; 73:812.

MELANIN BLEACH METHOD

FIXATION: 10% buffered neutral formalin.

SECTIONS: Paraffin, frozen, or celloidin; 6 to 12 micrometers.

SOLUTIONS

0.25% POTASSIUM PERMANGANATE SOLUTION

Potassium permanganate ....0.25 gm
Distilled water ....100.0 ml

5% OXALIC ACID SOLUTION

Oxalic acid ....5.0 gm
Distilled water ....100.0 ml

PROCEDURE

1. Deparaffinize and hydrate slides to distilled water.
2. Place in potassium permanganate solution for 5 minutes or longer.
3. Rinse carefully in distilled water.
4. Place in oxalic acid solution for 5 seconds or until the sections become clear.
5. Rinse carefully in distilled water.
6. Stain as indicated.

RESULTS

Melanin and lipofuscin pigments ....removed

ALTERNATE PROCEDURE

(Bleaching process accomplished when sectioning)

1. Float ribbon of paraffin sections or single celloidin or frozen sections onto the surface of a dish containing the potassium permanganate solution. Agitate gently and allow to remain for 5 minutes or longer.
2. Transfer individual sections through 2 changes of distilled water.
3. Float sections onto a dish containing the oxalic acid solution. Agitate gently and allow to remain until sections are clear.
4. Rinse sections in several changes of distilled water. Paraffin and frozen sections can then be picked up on premarked slides. Celloidin sections are held in distilled water until stained.
5. Dip slides into the heated water bath (42°C to 56°C), which contains gelatin.
6. Drain thoroughly.
7. Place slides on slide warming table (42°C to 48°C). Allow to dry overnight.
8. Paraffin sections are deparaffinized and hydrated to distilled water as usual. Mounted frozen sections are placed in distilled water. Stain as indicated.

RESULTS

Melanin and lipofuscin pigments ....removed

FONTANA-MASSON METHOD FOR ARGENTAFFIN GRANULES AND PIGMENTS

FIXATION: 10% buffered neutral formalin.

SECTIONS: Paraffin, 4 to 6 micrometers.

SOLUTIONS

10% SILVER NITRATE SOLUTION (Ch. 3)

FONTANA SILVER NITRATE STOCK SOLUTION

Silver nitrate, 10% ....95.0 ml
Ammonium hydroxide, concentrated, added **drop** by **drop** until the precipitate that forms clears.
Silver nitrate, 10%, added **drop** by **drop** until the solution becomes slightly cloudy.
Let stand overnight before using.

FONTANA SILVER NITRATE WORKING SOLUTION

Fontana silver nitrate solution, stock ....25.0 ml
Distilled water ....75.0 ml
Filter before using.

1% GOLD CHLORIDE STOCK SOLUTION (Ch. 3)

GOLD CHLORIDE WORKING SOLUTION

Gold chloride solution, 1% stock ....10.0 ml
Distilled water ....40.0 ml

5% SODIUM THIOSULFATE (HYPO) SOLUTION (Ch. 3)

NUCLEAR FAST RED SOLUTION (Ch. 3)

PROCEDURE

1. Deparaffinize and hydrate slides to distilled water.
2. Place slides in Fontana silver nitrate working solution and leave in a 37°C oven for 1 hour or until the sections are light brown. Check slides after 45 minutes, since oven temperatures vary. If the slides are very light brown remove from the oven and cool for 5 minutes.
3. Rinse in 3 changes of distilled water.
4. Tone in gold chloride working solution for 10 minutes.
5. Rinse in distilled water.
6. Place in sodium thiosulfate solution for 5 minutes.
7. Rinse in distilled water.
8. Counterstain with nuclear fast red solution for 5 minutes.
9. Rinse thoroughly in distilled water.

10. Dehydrate and clear in 95% ethyl alcohol, absolute ethyl alcohol, and xylene, 2 changes each, for 2 minutes each.
11. Mount with resinous medium.

RESULTS (See Fig. 20–2, page 200).

Argentaffin granules...black
Melanin[a] ....black
Nuclei and cytoplasm ....pink to red

[a]This procedure is non-specific for melanin, since other silver reducing substances will also stain.

REFERENCE

Masson P. Carcinoids and nerve hyperplasia of the appendicular mucosa. *Am J Pathol.* 1928;4:181.

CHURUKIAN-SCHENK METHOD FOR ARGYROPHIL GRANULES

FIXATION: 10% buffered neutral formalin.

SECTIONS: Paraffin, 4 to 6 micrometers.

SOLUTIONS
0.3% CITRIC ACID SOLUTION
Citric acid .... 0.3 gm
Sterile water .... 100.0 ml

ACIDIFIED WATER SOLUTION
Sterile water, irrigation .... 500.0 ml
Add sufficient quantity of the 0.3% citric acid solution to bring the pH to 4 or slightly above.

0.5 % SILVER NITRATE SOLUTION (FOR IMPREGNATION)
Silver nitrate .... 0.5 gm
Acidified water solution .... 100.0 ml
Preheat to 43°C a Coplin jar containing 30 to 40 ml of this silver solution.

DEVELOPER SOLUTION
Sodium sulfite, anhydrous .... 5.0 gm
Hydroquinone .... 1.0 gm
Sterile water .... 100.0 ml
Preheat to 56°C a Coplin jar containing 30 to 40 ml of the developer solution.

NUCLEAR FAST RED SOLUTION (Ch. 3)

PROCEDURE
1. Preheat two water baths, one to 43°C and one to 56°C.
2. Deparaffinize and hydrate slides to distilled water.
3. Place in acidified water solution for 3 minutes or longer.
4. Place in silver nitrate solution heated to 43°C for 2 minutes. Transfer slides and Coplin jar to heated 56°C water bath. Allow to remain for 2 hours. Save solution.
5. Flood slides with distilled water.
6. Place in preheated, 56°C, developer solution for 10 minutes. Save solution.
7. Rinse in 3 changes of distilled water.
8. Wash in running tap water for 3 minutes.
9. Rinse in 3 changes of distilled water.
10. Return slides to 0.5% silver nitrate solution and leave for 10 minutes.
11. Rinse in 3 changes of distilled water.
12. Return the slides to the preheated developer solution and leave for 10 minutes.
13. Rinse in 3 changes of distilled water.
14. Counterstain lightly in nuclear fast red solution for 3 minutes.
15. Rinse well in several changes of distilled water.

16. Dehydrate and clear through 95% ethyl alcohol, absolute ethyl alcohol, and xylene, 2 changes each, for 2 minutes each.
17. Mount with resinous medium.

RESULTS (See Fig. 20–3, page 200).

Argyrophil granules ....brown to black

Nuclei and cytoplasm ....red to pink

REFERENCE

Churukian CJ, Schenk EA. A modification of Pascual's argyrophil method. *J Histotechnol.* 1979;2:102.

AFIP METHOD FOR LIPOFUSCIN

FIXATION: 10% buffered neutral formalin.

SECTIONS: Paraffin, 6 micrometers.

SOLUTIONS

KINYOUN'S CARBOL FUCHSIN SOLUTION

Basic fuchsin ....4.0 gm
Phenol (carbolic acid) crystals, melted ....8.0 gm
Alcohol, 95% ethyl ....20.0 ml
Distilled water ....100.0 ml

Filter before using.

1% ACID ALCOHOL SOLUTION (Ch. 3)

PICRIC ACID SOLUTION, AQUEOUS (Ch. 3)

PROCEDURE

1. Deparaffinize and hydrate slides to distilled water.
2. Stain in Kinyoun's carbol fuchsin solution for 1 hour.
3. Rinse in several changes of distilled water.
4. Differentiate in acid alcohol solution, 5 or 6 dips or until the sections are pale pink.
5. Wash in running tap water for 5 minutes, then rinse in distilled water.
6. Counterstain in picric acid solution for approximately 1 minute.
7. Dehydrate and clear through 95% ethyl alcohol, absolute ethyl alcohol, and xylene, 2 changes each, for 2 minutes each.
8. Mount using resinous medium.

RESULTS

Lipofuscin ....red
Background ....yellow

HALL'S METHOD FOR BILIRUBIN

FIXATION: 10% buffered neutral formalin.

SECTIONS: Paraffin, 4 to 6 micrometers.

SOLUTIONS

10% FERRIC CHLORIDE SOLUTION

Ferric chloride .... 10.0 gm
Distilled water .... 100.0 ml

FOUCHET SOLUTION

Trichloroacetic acid .... 25.0 gm
Distilled water .... 100.0 ml
Mix thoroughly. Then add:
Ferric chloride, 10% solution .... 10.0 ml

VAN GIESON SOLUTION (Ch. 3)

PROCEDURE
1. Deparaffinize and hydrate slides to distilled water.
2. Place in Fouchet solution for 5 minutes.
3. Wash in running tap water for several minutes.
4. Rinse in distilled water.
5. Counterstain in van Gieson solution for 5 minutes.
6. Dehydrate and clear through 95% ethyl alcohol, absolute ethyl alcohol, and xylene, 2 changes each, for 2 minutes each.
7. Mount using resinous medium.

RESULTS

Bilirubin oxidized to biliverdin .... olive to emerald green
Collagen .... red
Muscle .... yellow

REFERENCE
Hall MJ. A staining reaction for bilirubin in sections of tissue. *Am J Clin Pathol.* 1960;34:313.

STABLE GMELIN REACTION

FIXATION: 10% buffered neutral formalin.

SECTIONS: Paraffin, 6 to 8 micrometers.

SOLUTIONS

0.5% BROMINE IN CARBON TETRACHLORIDE

Bromine ....0.25 ml
Carbon tetrachloride solution ....50.0 ml
Caution: a corrosive and irritant. Handle with care in a fume hood

PROCEDURE

1. Deparaffinize in three changes of xylene.
2. Dip in carbon tetrachloride.
3. Place in 0.5% bromine in carbon tetrachloride 10 minutes.
4. Air dry for 5 minutes.
5. Clear in two changes of xylene.
6. Mount with resinous medium.
7. Examine microscopically without delay, because the color tends to fade.

RESULTS

Bile pigments and hematoidin ....pale rose to dark red-purple to violet black.

REFERENCE

Lillie RD, Pizzolato P. A stable histochemical Gmelin reaction of bile pigments with dry bromine carbon tetrachloride solution. *J Histochem Cytochem.* 1967;15:600.

PROCEDURE FOR REMOVING HEMATIN (FORMALIN) AND MALARIA PIGMENTS

FIXATION: 10% buffered neutral formalin.

SECTIONS: Paraffin, 4 to 8 micrometers.

SOLUTION

SATURATED ALCOHOLIC PICRIC ACID SOLUTION

Picric acid ....9.0 gm
Alcohol, 95% ethyl ....100.0 ml

PROCEDURE

1. Deparaffinize and hydrate slides to distilled water.
2. Place in saturated alcoholic picric acid solution for 24 hours. However, if the specimens have been washed in running water for 16 hours prior to processing, the time is reduced to 5 to 10 minutes.
3. Wash thoroughly in running tap water until no yellow color remains.
4. Place in distilled water.
5. Stain as indicated.

RESULTS

Formalin and malaria pigments ....may be removed
Malaria parasites ....unchanged

PERLS IRON STAIN

FIXATION: 10% buffered neutral formalin.

SECTIONS: Paraffin, 4 to 8 micrometers.

SOLUTIONS

20% HYDROCHLORIC ACID

Hydrochloric acid ....20.0 ml
Distilled water ....80.0 ml

Add the acid to the water.

10% POTASSIUM FERROCYANIDE STOCK SOLUTION

Potassium ferrocyanide...10.0 gm
Distilled water ....100.0 ml

HYDROCHLORIC ACID-POTASSIUM FERROCYANIDE WORKING SOLUTION

Equal parts of 20% hydrochloric acid and 10% potassium ferrocyanide solution. Prepare just before use.

NUCLEAR FAST RED SOLUTION (Ch. 3)

PROCEDURE
1. Deparaffinize and hydrate slides to distilled water.
2. Place slides in freshly mixed hydrochloric acid-potassium ferrocyanide working solution for 30 minutes.
3. Rinse slides in distilled water.
4. Counterstain with nuclear fast red solution for 5 minutes.
5. Wash thoroughly in running tap water for 2 minutes.
6. Dehydrate and clear with 95% ethyl alcohol, absolute ethyl alcohol, and xylene, 2 changes each, for 2 minutes each.
7. Mount with resinous medium.

RESULTS   (See Fig. 20–4, page 201).

Hemosiderin and some oxides and salts of iron.................blue
Nuclei and cytoplasm ....pink to red

REFERENCES

Gomori G. Microchemical demonstration of iron. *Am J Pathol.* 1936;12:655.

Perls M. Nachweis von Eisenoxyd in gewissen pigmenten. *Virchows Archiv.* 1867;39:42.

MALLORY METHOD FOR IRON

FIXATION: 10% buffered neutral formalin.

SECTIONS: Paraffin, 4 to 6 micrometers.

SOLUTIONS

> 5% POTASSIUM FERROCYANIDE STOCK SOLUTION (Ch. 3)
>
> 5% HYDROCHLORIC ACID STOCK SOLUTION (Ch. 3)
>
> POTASSIUM FERROCYANIDE/HYDROCHLORIC ACID
> WORKING SOLUTION
>
> Potassium ferrocyanide solution, 5% stock .... 50.0 ml
> Hydrochloric acid solution, 5% stock .... 50.0 ml
>
> NUCLEAR FAST RED SOLUTION (Ch. 3)

PROCEDURE

1. Deparaffinize and hydrate slides to distilled water.
2. Place slides in potassium ferrocyanide/hydrochloric acid working solution for 10 minutes. Avoid any contact with metal.
3. Rinse slides in distilled water.
4. Counterstain with nuclear fast red solution for 5 minutes.
5. Wash thoroughly in running tap water for 2 minutes.
6. Dehydrate and clear with 95% ethyl alcohol, absolute ethyl alcohol, and xylene, 2 changes each, for 2 minutes each.
7. Mount with resinous medium.

RESULTS

> Hemosiderin and some oxides and salts of iron .... blue
> Nuclei and cytoplasm .... pink to red

REFERENCE
Mallory FB. Wright JH: *Pathological Technique*. Philadelphia, Pa: WB Saunders; 1924, p 207.

VON KOSSA METHOD FOR MINERALS

FIXATION: 10% buffered neutral formalin.

SECTIONS: Paraffin, 4 to 8 micrometers.

SOLUTIONS

5% SILVER NITRATE SOLUTION (Ch. 3)

PHOTOGRAPHIC DEVELOPER SOLUTION

Photographic developer (for B&W film or prints) .... 50.0 ml
Distilled water .... 50.0 ml

5% SODIUM THIOSULFATE (HYPO) SOLUTION Ch. 3)

NUCLEAR FAST RED SOLUTION (Ch. 3)

PROCEDURE

1. Deparaffinize and hydrate slides to water.
2. Place slides in 5% silver nitrate solution for 1 hour.
3. Rinse, with agitation, in 4 changes of distilled water.
4. Place in photographic developer solution for 2 minutes.
5. Rinse in 2 changes of distilled water.
6. Place in sodium thiosulfate solution for 5 minutes.
7. Wash in running tap water for 2 minutes.
8. Counterstain in nuclear fast red solution for 5 minutes.
9. Wash thoroughly in running tap water for 2 minutes.
10. Dehydrate and clear through 95% ethyl alcohol, absolute ethyl alcohol, and xylene, 2 changes each, for 2 minutes each.
11. Mount with resinous medium.

RESULTS   (See Fig. 20–5, page 201).

Bone and mineral salts (phosphates, carbonates, and oxalates)
  of calcium, iron, or other ions .... black deposits
Uric acid and its salts .... possibly, false-positive reactions
Nuclei and cytoplasm .... pink to red

REFERENCES

Gomori G. *Microscopic Histochemistry*. University of Chicago Press, Chicago, Ill: 1952:34.

Von Kossa J. Ueber die im Organismus kuenstlich erzeugbaren Verkakung. *Beitr Path Anat.* 1901;29:62.

ALIZARIN RED S PROCEDURE FOR CALCIUM

FIXATION: 10% buffered neutral formalin.

SECTIONS: Paraffin, 4 to 6 micrometers.

SOLUTIONS

ALIZARIN RED S SOLUTION

Alizarin red S ....2.0 gm
Distilled water ....100.0 ml
Adjust pH to 4.1 to 4.3 with ammonium hydroxide added drop by drop. Stir constantly.

ACETONE

ACETONE-XYLENE SOLUTION

Acetone ....50.0 ml
Xylene ....50.0 ml

PROCEDURE

1. Deparaffinize and hydrate slides to distilled water.
2. Place in alizarin red S solution for 30 seconds to 5 minutes.
3. Examine microscopically. When red-orange color appears, shake off excess stain.
4. Do not counterstain.
5. Dehydrate and clear rapidly through acetone, acetone-xylene solution, then xylene.
6. Mount using resinous medium.

RESULTS

Most calcium salts ....birefringent red precipitates
Calcium oxalate ....no reaction

REFERENCE
McGee-Russell SM. Histochemical methods for calcium. *J Histochem Cytochem.* 1958;6:22.

RHODANINE METHOD FOR COPPER

FIXATION: 10% buffered neutral formalin.

SECTIONS: Paraffin, 4 to 6 micrometers.

SOLUTIONS

0.2% RHODANINE STOCK SOLUTION

5-(p-dimethylaminobenzylidine) rhodanine ....0.2 gm
Alcohol, absolute, ethyl ....100.0 ml

ACETATE BUFFER SOLUTION, pH 8.0 - pH 8.3

Formalin, 40% ....5.0 ml
Sodium acetate ....20.0 gm
Distilled water ....1000.0 ml

RHODANINE WORKING SOLUTION

Rhodanine, 0.2% stock ....3.0 ml
Acetate buffer solution ....50.0 ml

MAYER'S HEMATOXYLIN SOLUTION (Ch. 9)

PROCEDURE

1. Deparaffinize and hydrate slides to distilled water.
2. Place in rhodanine working solution at 37°C for 18 hours.
3. Rinse in 3 changes of acetate buffer solution, pH 8.0 to pH 8.3.
4. Counterstain in Mayer's hematoxylin solution for 10 minutes.
5. Rinse in 3 changes of acetate buffer solution, pH 8.0 to pH 8.3.
6. Dehydrate and clear through 95% ethyl alcohol, absolute ethyl alcohol, and xylene, 2 changes each, for 2 minutes each.
7. Mount with resinous medium.

RESULTS (See Fig. 20–6, page 201).

Copper ....red
Nuclei ....blue

REFERENCE

Lindquist RR. Studies on the pathogenesis of hepatolenticular degeneration, II: cytochemical methods for the location of copper. *Arch Pathol.* 1969;87:370.

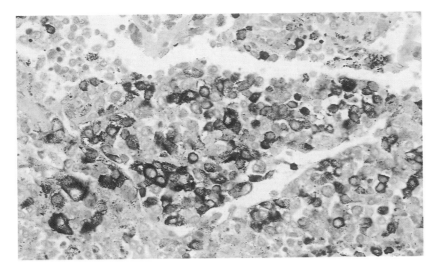

Fig. 20–1.
Warthin-Starry
pH. 3.2 .
Lymph Node with
malignant
melanoma.

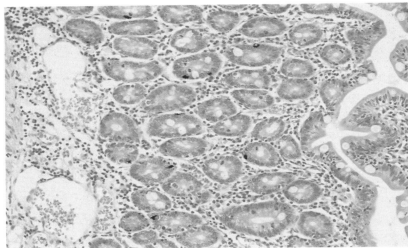

Fig. 20–2.
Fontana-Masson.
Endocrine cells in
ileal mucosa.

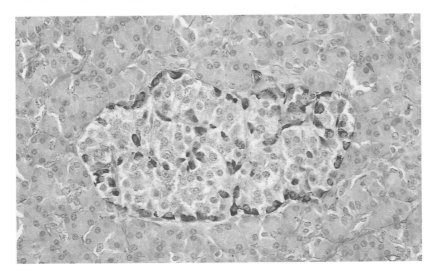

Fig. 20–3.
Churukian-
Schenk.
Pancreatic islet.

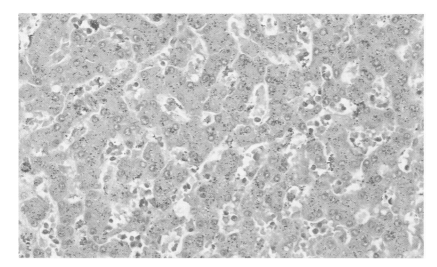

Fig. 20–4.
Perls iron.
Siderosis. Liver.

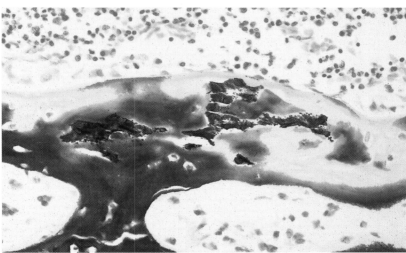

Fig. 20–5.
Von Kossa. Bone

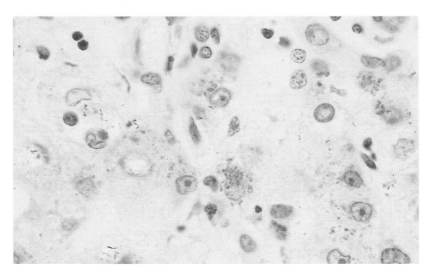

Fig. 20–6.
Rhodanine.
Copper granules
in liver cell
cytoplasm.

AFIP Laboratory Methods in Histotechnology

CHAPTER 21

BACTERIA, FUNGI, AND OTHER MICROORGANISMS

Jacquelyn B. Arrington

Special staining techniques that demonstrate infectious organisms in paraffin sections and smears are an invaluable diagnostic tool for pathologists. The principles upon which the various techniques are based are discussed in this chapter. Descriptions of a number of microorganisms are presented along with the stains that may be used to demonstrate them.

BACTERIA

Some bacteria are visible in hematoxylin and eosin preparations using high-dry or oil-immersion light microscopy. Greater sensitivity to their presence and specificity in their identification are achieved with special stains, as described in this section.

I. Gram-negative and Gram-positive Bacteria

Various Gram stains are available that selectively stain Gram-negative and Gram positive bacteria. Although Gram stains may require different dyes, dye concentrations, and decolorizers, the staining procedures do not vary significantly. The Gram stains used most often at the AFIP are the Brown and Hopps stain and the Brown and Brenn stain. The Brown and Hopps stain is preferred for its consistency in results.

The basic steps involved in most Gram stains follow:
1. Flood tissue with primary stain (usually crystal violet). Rinse.
2. Flood tissue with iodine to form a dye lake between crystal violet and gram positive organisms. Rinse.
3. Decolorize. Gram-positive organisms, if present, will retain color. Rinse.
4. Flood tissue with counterstain (usually basic fuchsin). Rinse.
5. Differentiate. Gram-negative organisms, if present, will retain stain. Rinse.
6. Stain background.
7. Differentiate.
8. Use acetone/xylene solutions and xylene to dehydrate and clear.

Selected Gram-negative and Gram-positive bacteria are described below. Other useful stains are also provided.

NAME	DESCRIPTION	OTHER STAINS

GRAM-POSITIVE BACTERIA (BLUE TO VIOLET)

NAME	DESCRIPTION	OTHER STAINS
Corynebacterium sp	Rods	PAS
Listeria sp	Rods	
Pneumococcus sp	Pairs or chains of cocci	H&E, PAS
Staphylococcus sp	Clusters of cocci	PAS
Streptococcus sp	Round or elliptical, chains or pairs of cocci	

GRAM-NEGATIVE BACTERIA (RED)

NAME	DESCRIPTION	OTHER STAINS
Brucella sp	Rods or cocci, depending on species	H&E
Helicobacter sp (*Campylobacter*)	Curved rods, gull-shaped forms	H&E, Giemsa, PAS WS (pH 4.0)
Escherichia coli	Single, paired, or long filaments	
Fusobacterium sp	Paired, large slender rods	
Hemophilus sp	Cocci with capsules	
Klebsiella sp	Single or paired encapsulated rods	Giemsa
Neisseria sp	Gram-negative cocci	MGP
Pasteurella sp	Short rods or cocci, pleomorphic	Giemsa
Proteus sp	Rods. Forms may vary among species.	
Pseudomonas sp	Short rods	
Salmonella sp	Paired or single small rods	H&E
Shigella sp	Blunt rods	H&E
Vibrio sp	Curved rods with single polar flagellum	

II. Acid-fast Bacteria

Some species of bacteria maintain carbofuchsin staining after being treated with acid decolorizers. The organisms are said to be acid-fast. Included in this group are the *Mycobacterium* species and *Nocardia asteroides*. Staining times, decolorizers, and deparaffinization steps may vary among the several procedures for acid-fast organisms. The primary stains and counterstains, however, remain the same.

A general procedure for acid-fast organisms follows:
1. After deparaffinization, stain section with carbofuchsin. Rinse.
2. Decolorize. Acid-fast organisms will retain their bright red color, and the background will be clear. Sections will be pale pink and transparent. Rinse.
3. Counterstain with methylene blue. Note: If the counterstain is too dark, acid fast organisms may not be visible. A counterstain that is too light, however, will not adequately demonstrate the tissue components.
4. Dehydrate, clear, and mount.

SELECTED ACID-FAST BACTERIA

NAME	DESCRIPTION	PREFERRED STAIN
Mycobacterium sp		
M leprae	Rods	Fite
M tuberculosis	Rods	Ziehl-Neelsen
M avium intracellulare	Rods	Ziehl-Neelsen and PAS
Nocardia asteroides	Delicate filaments	Coates Fite

III. Bacteria Stained by Silver Impregnation

Bacteria may also be demonstrated by silver impregnation. This technique involves exposure of sections to silver solutions. The organisms are blackened when the silver is reduced to its metallic state. Crucial to this technique is the staining of the bacteria while maintaining a clear background, since silver may also stain other tissue elements. Spirochetes and the bacillus thought to cause cat-scratch disease are well demonstrated by Warthin-Starry. Some bacteria are more easily seen by this technique because the coating of silver makes them appear larger than with other stains, e.g. *Helicobacter (Campylobacter) pyloris*. Many bacteria are stained by the Warthin-Starry pH 4.0 technique. Therefore, if organisms are detected, specific identification usually requires other special staining techniques.

FUNGI

Fungi are plants that do not have stems, leaves, or roots and lack chlorophyll. Their cell walls may contain chitin, which is, generally speaking, argyrophilic and PAS-positive (diastase resistant). The structure of fungi varies according to classification. They may be filamentous, yeasts, yeast-like, or pleomorphic. Filamentous fungi produce long structures called hyphae, which may or may not be segmented. Yeasts reproduce by budding. Yeastlike fungi produce long pseudohyphae. Pleomorphism is a phenomenon whereby fungi change their form with changes in temperature and location such as from growth in the body to growth in a culture medium.

Disease-causing fungi may infect humans superficially, e.g. in the skin and the nails, or they may be systemic. Opportunistic fungi become pathogenic when the patient's immune system is impaired.

SELECTED FUNGI AND STAINING TECHNIQUES

NAME	DESCRIPTION	STAINS
Actinomyces sp	Delicate, branching filaments <1 micrometer in diameter	GMS Gram-positive Giemsa, PAS
Nocardia asteroides	Narrow, delicate threads, 0.5-1.0 micrometer that branch at right angles	GMS Gram-positive Giemsa
Aspergillus fumigatis	Y-shaped, branched with segmented hyphae	GMS Gridley Fungus PAS
Dermatophytes	Branching hyphae that may break into chains called arthroconidia	GMS Gram-positive Giemsa
Histoplasma capsulatum	Small, ovoid yeast cells, 2-4 micrometers in diameter	GMS Gridley Fungus
Blastomycetes	Budding round-to-oval yeastlike cells with thick walls	GMS, PAS Gridley Fungus
Candida albicans	Branching septate hyphae, chains of budding cells, hyphae may bear spores	GMS, H&E, PAS Gram-positive Gridley Fungus
Cryptococcus neoformans	Budding yeast cells with thin walls, 2-20 micrometers in diameter	Mucicarmine Gram-positive AB-PAS, GMS Gridley Fungus Colloidal Iron

The fungi listed above stain with the Grocott's methenamine silver nitrate stain (GMS), which blackens their walls. Care must be taken to demonstrate the fungi while discouraging background staining and silver precipitate formation.

AFIP Laboratory Methods in Histotechnology

VIRUSES

Viruses are minute, obligate intracellular parasites that cannot be seen by light microscopy. Aggregates of viral particles, however, may be demonstrated in paraffin sections. These particles found in host cells are called viral inclusion bodies. The individual particles that form the cellular inclusions are referred to as elementary bodies.

There are some inclusion bodies that may be observed with the H&E stain. Viral infection may also be detected by staining the viral antigen, e.g., with immunohistochemical techniques. The hepatitis B surface antigen is demonstrated by orcein or aldehyde fuchsin.

RICKETTSIAE

Rickettsiae are also obligate intracellular parasites. These parasites are carried by ticks, mites, or lice and appear in paraffin sections as small coccobacilli. Rickettsiae are responsible for tick-borne diseases such as Rocky Mountain spotted fever and typhus. The elementary bodies of rickettsiae stain pale blue to violet with H&E and reddish purple with Giemsa and are gram-negative.

PARASITES

Included in this category are a variety of organisms ranging from one-celled protozoans to grossly visible worms. The malarial protozoan can be seen with the Giemsa stain. Basophilic and acidophilic tissue elements are stained simultaneously. The azure eosin compounds used to prepare the Giemsa solution readily stain erythrocytes that are infected by the malarial parasite. Optimum staining results require a controlled pH.

Pneumocystis carinii is an opportunistic organism that flourishes in the lungs of persons with immune deficiency. It is a small ovoid organism usually demonstrated by the GMS technique. After silver impregnation, the walls are blackened. The parasite is then observed against a light-green background.

Other parasites in the Platyhelminthes and nematode groups may be demonstrated by H&E, Giemsa, and PAS methods. The Russell-Movat pentachrome procedure is excellent for the demonstration of the morphology of animal parasites. Structures may be clearly identified according to staining results. The Movat method is presented in the chapter on connective tissues.

MODIFIED ORCEIN METHOD
FOR HEPATITIS B SURFACE ANTIGEN

FIXATION: 10% buffered neutral formalin or formol saline.

SECTIONS: Paraffin, 6 micrometers.

SOLUTIONS

0.15% POTASSIUM PERMANGANATE SOLUTION

Potassium permanganate ....0.15 gm
Distilled water ....100.0 ml
Before using, add 0.15 ml of concentrated sulfuric acid.

1.5% OXALIC ACID SOLUTION (Ch. 3)

ORCEIN SOLUTION

Orcein (preferably BDH)[a] ....1.0 gm
Alcohol, 70% ethyl ....100.0 ml
Hydrochloric acid, concentrated ....1.0 ml

Let age at room temperature for 5 to 7 days. Filter and refrigerate for 1 day before using. This will eliminate some background staining. Store solution in refrigerator.

PROCEDURE

1. Deparaffinize and hydrate to distilled water.
2. Place in 0.15% potassium permanganate solution for 5 minutes.
3. Rinse in 2 changes of distilled water.
4. Place in 1.5% oxalic acid solution until sections are colorless, usually 10 to 15 seconds.
5. Wash gently in tap water for 1 minute.
6. Rinse in distilled water, 2 changes by pouring on and off.
7. Rinse in 2 changes of 95% ethyl alcohol.
8. Stain in orcein solution overnight.
9. Rinse in 2 changes each of 95% ethyl alcohol and absolute alcohol.
10. Clear in 3 changes of xylene.
11. Mount with resinous medium.

RESULTS

There is dark-brown staining of all or part of the cytoplasm of liver cells that have "ground-glass" cytoplasm with the hematoxylin and eosin stain.[b] Positively stained cytoplasm corresponds to localization of hepatitis B surface antigen as determined by immunofluorescence and immune electron microscopy. Orcein also stains elastic tissue and copper-associated protein (metallothionine). The latter appears as brown granules.

aArtificial dyes will not render desired results. ORCEIN, Product No. 34063, manufactured by British Drug House (BDH) Chemical Ltd., Poole, England. U.S.A. distributor: Gallard-Schlesinger, Chemical Mfg. Corp. Carle Place, N.Y. 11514.

b"Ground-glass" cells can also be stained by the aldehyde-fuchsin stain for elastic tissue, as well as Victoria blue.

REFERENCES

Deodhar KP. Orcein staining of hepatitis B antigen in paraffin sections of liver biopsies. *J Clin Pathol.* 1975;28:66.

Shikata T. Staining methods of Australia antigen in paraffin sections. *Jpn J Exp Med.* 1974;44:25.

VICTORIA BLUE (TANAKA) METHOD
FOR HEPATITIS B SURFACE ANTIGEN

FIXATION: 10% buffered neutral formalin.

SECTIONS: Paraffin, 6 micrometers.

SOLUTIONS

VICTORIA BLUE SOLUTION

Dextrine	0.5 gm
Victoria blue	2.0 gm
Resorcinol	4.0 gm

Gradually heat. Bring to boiling. Add:
Boiling ferric chloride solution, 29% ....25.0 ml

0.3% POTASSIUM PERMANGANATE STOCK SOLUTION (Ch. 3)

0.3% SULFURIC ACID STOCK SOLUTION (Ch. 3)

POTASSIUM PERMANGANATE-SULFURIC ACID WORKING SOLUTION

Stock 0.3% potassium permanganate solution ....50.0 ml
Stock 0.3% sulfuric acid solution ....50.0 ml
Make fresh.

4% SODIUM BISULFITE SOLUTION

Sodium bisulfite	4.0 gm
Distilled water	100.0 ml

Make fresh.

NUCLEAR FAST RED SOLUTION (Ch. 3)

PROCEDURE

1. Deparaffinize and hydrate to distilled water.
2. Place in potassium permanganate-sulfuric acid working solution for 5 minutes.
3. Place in 4% sodium bisulfite solution for 1 minute.
4. Wash in running water.
5. Rinse in 70% ethyl alcohol for a few minutes.
6. Stain in Victoria blue solution for 24 hours or longer.[a]
7. Differentiate in 70% ethyl alcohol for 3-5 minutes or longer, until the background has become completely decolorized.[b]
8. Wash in running water for a few minutes.
9. Counterstain in nuclear fast red solution for 5 minutes.
10. Wash in running water for 5 minutes.
11. Dehydrate and clear through 2 changes each of 95% ethyl alcohol, absolute ethyl alcohol, and xylene, 2 minutes each.
12. Mount with resinous medium.

RESULTS

Hepatitis B surface antigen .... blue
Lipofuscin, mast cells, elastin, mucin .... blue
Nuclei and cytoplasm .... red
Bile pigment .... red
Hemosiderin .... pale blue
Copper-associated protein .... blue

[a]Proper staining may require 1 day to 1 week.

[b]Proper differentiation may require 3 minutes to 24 hours.

REFERENCE

Tanaka AB. Victoria blue-nuclear fast red stain for HBs antigen detection in paraffin sections. *Acta Pathol Jpn.* 1981;31:93.

GAFFNEY'S ONE-HOUR GIEMSA

FIXATION: 10% buffered neutral formalin.

SECTIONS: Paraffin, 4 to 6 micrometers.

SOLUTIONS

AZURE II-EOSIN SOLUTION

Place a few sterile glass beads into a 1,000-ml amber bottle.
Add azure II eosin ....1.3 gm
    Glycerin ....80.0 ml
Heat at 56°C for 2 hours. Mix and cool. Add:
    Methyl alcohol, absolute ....170.0 ml
    Acetone ....170.0 ml

MAY-GRÜNWALD STAIN SOLUTION

Combine in a 1,000-ml flask:
    May-Grünwald stain ....0.15 gm
    Methyl alcohol, absolute ....290.0 ml
    Acetone ....290.0 ml

STOCK GIEMSA SOLUTION

Combine the above solutions—azure II-eosin solution and the May-Grünwald solution—and label as stock.

ACETIC WATER SOLUTION (pH 4.7)

    Acetic acid, glacial ....1 drop
    Distilled water..1000.0 ml

GIEMSA WORKING SOLUTION

    Giemsa solution (stock) ....10.0 ml
    Acetic water solution ....50.0 ml
Make fresh. Discard after use.

PROCEDURE
    1.   Deparaffinize and hydrate to distilled water.
    2.   Stain in freshly prepared Giemsa working solution for 1 hour.
    3.   Check microscopically.[a]
    4.   Dehydrate in 3 changes of absolute alcohol.
    5.   Clear in xylene, 3 changes.
    6.   Mount with resinous medium.

RESULTS

Cytoplasm	pink
Nuclei	blue
Erythrocytes	red
Mast-cell granules	purple
Bacteria	blue
Malaria parasites	blue

[a]If sections are blue and are not differentially stained, the acetic water solution may be too old. Repeat the procedure with fresh acetic water solution.

REFERENCES

Lillie RD. *Histopathologic Technic and Practical Histochemistry.* New York, NY: McGraw-Hill; 1976:193.

Sheehan DC. *Theory and Practice of Histotechnology.* Columbus, Ohio: Battelle Press; 1980:55.

Strumia MM. A rapid universal blood stain. *J Lab Clin Med.* 1936;21:930.

MODIFIED WARTHIN-STARRY METHOD (pH 4.0) FOR SPIROCHETES AND OTHER MICROORGANISMS

FIXATION: 10% buffered neutral formalin.

SECTIONS: Paraffin, 6 micrometers.

SOLUTIONS

1% CITRIC ACID SOLUTION

Citric acid .... 1.0 gm
Distilled water .... 100.0 ml

ACIDULATED WATER SOLUTION

Sterile water .... 1000.0 ml
Add enough 1% citric acid solution to reach a pH 4.0.

1% SILVER IMPREGNATING SOLUTION

Silver nitrate .... 1.0 gm
Acidulated water .... 100.0 ml

2% SILVER NITRATE SOLUTION

Silver nitrate .... 2.0 gm
Acidulated water .... 100.0 ml
Place flask in a flotation bath set at 54°C.

5% GELATIN SOLUTION

Gelatin .... 5.0 gm
Acidulated water .... 100.0 ml
Place flask in a flotation bath set at 54°C.

0.15% PYROCATECHOL SOLUTION

Pyrocatechol .... 0.15 gm
Acidulated water .... 100.0 ml
Place flask in a flotation bath set at 54°C.

DEVELOPING SOLUTION

Silver nitrate solution, 2% .... 1.5 ml
Gelatin solution, 5% .... 3.75 ml
Pyrocatechol solution, 0.15% .... 2.0 ml

Just before use combine in a small beaker in the order given. Mix the silver nitrate solution and the gelatin solution thoroughly before adding the pyrocatechol solution.

PROCEDURE

1. Deparaffinize and hydrate to distilled water.
2. Impregnate in 1% silver nitrate solution at 43°C for 30 minutes.
3. Place slides on staining rack using glass rods. Flood with the developing solution. Allow color to develop to yellow brown.
4. Wash quickly and thoroughly in hot tap water to stop reaction.
5. Dehydrate and clear through 95% ethyl alcohol, absolute ethyl alcohol, and xylene, 2 changes each, 2 minutes each.
6. Mount with resinous medium.

RESULTS

Background ....tan to yellow
Spirochetes and other microorganisms ....black

REFERENCES

Allen TC, Luna LG, Wear DJ. Modified Warthin-Starry technique. *AFIP Letter.* 1986;144:3.

Kerr DA. Improved Warthin-Starry method of staining spirochetes in tissue sections. *Am J Clin Pathol.* 1938;8:63.

THOMAS METHOD FOR MALARIAL PARASITES

FIXATION: Any well-fixed tissue.

TECHNIQUE: Paraffin, 6 micrometers.

SOLUTIONS

PHLOXINE B SOLUTION

Phloxine B	0.5 gm
Distilled water	100.0 ml
Acetic acid, glacial	1.0 ml

METHYLENE BLUE-AZURE B SOLUTION

Methylene blue	0.25 gm
Azure B	0.25 gm
Borax	0.25 gm
Distilled water	100.0 ml

0.2% GLACIAL ACETIC ACID SOLUTION (Ch. 3)

PROCEDURE
1. Deparaffinize and hydrate to distilled to water.
2. Stain in phloxine B solution for 2 minutes.
3. Rinse in distilled water.
4. Stain in methylene blue-azure B solution for 1 minute.
5. Differentiate with glacial acetic acid solution.
6. Complete differentiation in 95% alcohol, 3 changes.
7. Dehydrate in absolute alcohol, then clear in xylene, 2 changes each.
8. Mount with resinous medium.

RESULTS

Nuclei	blue
Plasma cell cytoplasm	blue
Malarial parasites	blue
Erythrocytes	pink
Other tissue elements	rose to red

REFERENCE

Thomas JT. Phloxine-methylene blue staining of formalin-fixed tissue. *Stain Technol.* 1953;28:311.

FITE'S METHOD FOR ACID-FAST BACTERIA

FIXATION: 10% buffered neutral formalin.

SECTIONS: Paraffin, 6 micrometers.

SOLUTIONS

XYLENE-PEANUT OIL SOLUTION

Peanut oil .... 1 part
Xylene .... 2 parts

ZIEHL-NEELSEN CARBOL-FUCHSIN SOLUTION

Phenol crystals, melted .... 2.5 ml
Alcohol, absolute, ethyl .... 5.0 ml
Basic fuchsin .... 0.5 gm
Distilled water .... 50.0 ml
Filter before use.

1% ACID ALCOHOL SOLUTION[a] (Ch. 3)

METHYLENE BLUE STOCK SOLUTION (Ch. 3)

METHYLENE BLUE WORKING SOLUTION

Methylene blue solution, stock .... 10.0 ml
Tap water .... 90.0 ml

PROCEDURE
1. Deparaffinize slides through 2 changes of xylene-peanut oil solution for 12 minutes each.
2. Allow slides to air-dry for 15 minutes. The remaining oil film will help to prevent shrinkage and injury to sections.[b]
3. Stain in filtered carbol-fuchsin solution for 30 minutes.
4. Wash in tap water for 10 minutes.
5. Differentiate slides in 1% acid alcohol solution until sections are pale pink.
6. Wash in running for 3 minutes.
7. Counterstain in methylene blue working solution for 30 seconds to 1 minute.
8. Rinse off excess methylene blue working solution with tap water.[c]
9. Dehydrate the slides quickly through 2 changes each of 95% and absolute ethyl alcohol. Do not leave slides in alcohol.
10. Clear in 2 changes of xylene, 2 minutes each.
11. Mount with resinous medium.

RESULTS (See Figs. 21–1, page 233).

Lepra and other acid-fast bacilli[d]. .... red
Nocardia filaments .... red
Background .... pale blue

a1% acid alcohol is preferred to the 1% sulfuric acid water used as the decolorizer in the original procedure.

bThe peanut-oil film is more evenly distributed when slides are air-dried rather than blotted. Blotting slides may also cause damage to the sections.

cIf methylene blue staining is too light, other tissue elements may be difficult to identify. Sections that are too lightly stained with methylene blue may become colorless after rinsing with water. A deep sky blue background will adequately stain other tissue elements without obscuring the red acid-fast bacilli.

dAlthough other acid-fast bacilli are demonstrated, this stain is used primarily for the demonstration of lepra bacilli.

REFERENCE

Fite GL, Cambre PJ, Turner MH. Procedure for demonstrating lepra bacilli in paraffin sections. *Arch Pathol.* 1947;43:624.

ZIEHL-NEELSEN METHOD FOR ACID-FAST BACTERIA
AFIP Modification

FIXATION: Any well-fixed tissue.

SECTIONS: Paraffin, 4 to 6 micrometers.

SOLUTIONS

ZIEHL-NEELSEN CARBOL-FUCHSIN SOLUTION

Phenol crystals, melted ....2.5 ml
Alcohol, absolute, ethyl ....5.0 ml
Basic fuchsin..0.5 gm
Distilled water ....50.0 ml
Filter before use.

1% ACID ALCOHOL SOLUTION (Ch. 3)

METHYLENE BLUE STOCK SOLUTION (Ch. 3)

METHYLENE BLUE WORKING SOLUTION (Ch. 3)

PROCEDURE

1. Deparaffinize and hydrate to distilled water.
2. Stain sections with freshly filtered carbol-fuchsin solution for 30 minutes.
3. Wash well in running tap water.
4. Decolorize with 1% acid alcohol solution until sections are pale pink.[a]
5. Wash thoroughly in running water for 8 minutes.
6. Counterstain by dipping one slide at a time in methylene blue working solution.[b] Sections should be pale blue.[c] Overcounterstaining will mask the bacilli.
7. Wash with tap water, then with distilled water.[d]
8. Dehydrate quickly in 95% ethyl alcohol and absolute ethyl alcohol, 2 changes each, clear in 2 changes of xylene, 2 minutes each.
9. Mount with resinous medium.

RESULTS   (See Fig. 21-2, page 233).

Acid-fast bacilli ....bright red
Erythrocytes ....yellow orange
Other tissue elements ....blue

[a]The preferred decolorizer is 1% acid alcohol solution. 1% sulfuric acid solution was used in the original procedure.

[b]Slides may be counterstained in groups rather than by dipping one at a time as stated in the original procedure.

[c]Avoid insufficient counterstaining with methylene blue working solution, since other tissue structures may not be demonstrated.

[d]Rinsing in tap water differentiates methylene blue working solution. It is possible to wash out too much of the counterstain so that the background will be understained.

ACID-FAST STAIN
(Modified for microwave staining)

FIXATION: 10% buffered neutral formalin

SECTIONS: Paraffin, 4 to 8 micrometers

SOLUTIONS

ZIEHL-NEELSEN CARBOL-FUCHSIN SOLUTION

Phenol crystals, melted .... 2.5 ml
Alcohol, absolute, ethyl .... 5.0 ml
Basic fuchsin .... 0.5 gm
Distilled water .... 50.0 ml

Filter before use.

1% ACID ALCOHOL SOLUTION (Ch. 3)

METHYLENE BLUE STOCK SOLUTION (Ch. 3)

METHYLENE BLUE WORKING SOLUTION (Ch. 3)

PROCEDURE

1. Deparaffinize and hydrate slides to distilled water.
2. Place slides in carbol fuchsin and microwave with thermal probe set to cut off at 200°F.
3. Allow slides to stand in warm solution for 5 minutes.
4. Rinse in running tap water.
5. Dip in acid alcohol solution and then rinse in tap water repeatedly until the sections are pale pink.
6. Stain in working solution of methylene blue for 30 seconds.
7. Rinse in tap water.
8. Dehydrate, clear, and mount in resinous medium.

RESULTS

Acid-fast bacilli .... red
Background .... blue

REFERENCE

Hafiz S, Spencer RC, Lee M, Gooch H, Duerden BI. Use of microwaves for acid and alcohol fast staining. *J Clin Pathol.* 1985;38:1073.

BROWN-HOPPS GRAM STAIN
AFIP Modification

FIXATION: 10% buffered neutral formalin.

SECTIONS: Paraffin, 6 micrometers.

SOLUTIONS

1% CRYSTAL VIOLET SOLUTION (Ch. 3)

1% BASIC FUCHSIN SOLUTION (Ch. 3)

GRAM'S IODINE SOLUTION (Ch. 3)

GALLEGO'S DIFFERENTIATING SOLUTION

Distilled water .... 100.0 ml
Formalin, 37-40% solution .... 2.0 ml
Acetic acid, glacial .... 1.0 ml

PICRIC ACID-ACETONE SOLUTION (Ch. 3)

ACETONE

ACETONE-XYLENE SOLUTION (Ch. 3)

PROCEDURE
1. Deparaffinize and hydrate slides to distilled water.
2. Place in 1% crystal violet solution for 1 minute.[a]
3. Rinse in tap water.
4. Place in Gram's iodine solution for 1 minute.
5. Rinse in tap water.
6. Decolorize in acetone until background is clear.
7. Immediately wash in tap water.
8. Place in 1% basic fuchsin solution for 5 minutes.[b]
9. Rinse in tap water.
10. Place in Gallego's differentiating solution, 2 changes, 1 minute each.
11. Rinse in tap water.
12. Transfer to a staining dish.[c]
13. Treat with acetone for 30 seconds.
14. Place in picric acid-acetone solution for 2-3 minutes.[d]
15. Place in acetone-xylene solution for 2 changes.
16. Clear in xylene, 2 changes.
17. Mount with resinous medium.

RESULTS

Gram-positive bacteria .... blue
Gram-negative bacteria .... red
Background .... yellow

[a]A staining rack is used for staining the slides in steps 2 through 11.

[b]The original procedure called for a 0.1% basic fuchsin solution.

[c]Use a staining dish for steps 12 through 16.

[d]Picric acid-acetone has been substituted for the tartrazine counterstain used in the original procedure.

REFERENCE
Brown RC, Hopps HC. Staining of bacteria in tissue sections: Reliable Gram stain method. *Am J Clin Pathol.* 1973;60:234.

BROWN AND BRENN GRAM STAIN
AFIP Modification

FIXATION: 10% buffered neutral formalin.

SECTIONS: Paraffin, 6 micrometers.

SOLUTIONS

1% CRYSTAL VIOLET SOLUTION (Ch. 3)

5% SODIUM BICARBONATE SOLUTION (Ch. 3)

GRAM'S IODINE SOLUTION (Ch. 3)

0.25% BASIC FUCHSIN STOCK SOLUTION (Ch. 3)

BASIC FUCHSIN WORKING SOLUTION

Basic fuchsin, stock .... 10.0 ml
Distilled water .... 90.0 ml

ACETONE[a]

PICRIC ACID-ACETONE SOLUTION

Picric acid .... 0.1 gm
Acetone .... 100.0 ml

ACETONE-XYLENE SOLUTION

Acetone .... 50.0 ml
Xylene .... 50.0 ml

PROCEDURE
1. Deparaffinize and hydrate to distilled water.
2. Place slides on staining rack. Pour on 1 ml (20 drops) of crystal violet solution and add 5 drops of 5% sodium bicarbonate solution for 1 minute. Agitate gently. Solution may be mixed just before use.
3. Rinse in tap water.
4. Flood with Gram's iodine solution for 1 minute.
5. Rinse in tap water.
6. Decolorize with acetone.
7. Rinse in tap water.
8. Flood with basic fuchsin working solution for 1 minute. Rinse.
9. Place slides in Coplin jar in tap water.[b]
10. Dip individually in acetone to start reaction.
11. Differentiate each slide immediately with picric acid-acetone solution until sections are yellowish pink.

12. Rinse quickly in acetone, then in acetone-xylene solution.
13. Clear in 2 changes of xylene and mount with resinous medium.

RESULTS

Gram-positive bacteria .... blue
Gram-negative bacteria .... red
Filaments of Nocardia and Actinomyces .... blue
Nuclei .... red
Other tissue elements .... yellow

[a]Originally, ethyl ether-acetone solution was used to decolorize sections that had first been blotted dry. Because the use of ethyl ether has been discouraged in laboratories for safety reasons, acetone is now used as the decolorizer.

[b]Slides are held in water prior to placement in acetone. Slides are no longer blotted dry before acetone.

REFERENCE
Brown JH, Brenn L. Bulletin Johns Hopkins Hospital. 1931;48:69.

GROCOTT'S METHENAMINE SILVER NITRATE METHOD FOR FUNGI (GMS)

FIXATION: 10% buffered neutral formalin.

SECTIONS: Paraffin, 6 micrometers.

SOLUTIONS

4% CHROMIC ACID SOLUTION (Ch. 3)

5% SILVER NITRATE SOLUTION (Ch. 3)

3% METHENAMINE SOLUTION (Ch. 3)

5% BORAX SOLUTION (Ch. 3)

METHENAMINE-SILVER NITRATE STOCK SOLUTION

Silver nitrate, 5% solution	5.0 ml
Methenamine, 3% solution	100.0 ml

METHENAMINE-SILVER NITRATE WORKING SOLUTION

Methenamine-silver nitrate solution, stock	25.0 ml
Distilled water[a]	25.0 ml
Borax, 5% solution	2.0 ml

Prepare fresh prior to use. Do not use if cloudy.

1% SODIUM BISULFITE SOLUTION (Ch. 3)

0.1% GOLD CHLORIDE SOLUTION (Ch. 3)

5% SODIUM THIOSULFATE (HYPO) SOLUTION (Ch. 3)

0.2% LIGHT GREEN STOCK SOLUTION (Ch. 3)

LIGHT GREEN WORKING SOLUTION

Light green, stock	10.0 ml
Distilled water	50.0 ml

PROCEDURE: Use acid-cleaned glassware.
1. Deparaffinize and hydrate to distilled water.
2. Oxidize in fresh 4% chromic acid solution for 1 hour.
3. Wash in tap water for a few seconds.

4. Place in sodium bisulfite solution for 1 minute to remove any residual chromic acid solution.
5. Wash in running water for 5 to 10 minutes.
6. Rinse with 3 or 4 changes of distilled water.
7. Place in freshly mixed methenamine-silver nitrate working solution in oven at 58° to 60°C for 50 to 60 minutes.[b]
8. Rinse in 6 changes of distilled water.
9. Tone in gold chloride solution for 2 to 5 minutes.
10. Rinse in distilled water.
11. Place in sodium thiosulfate solution for 2 to 5 minutes.
12. Wash thoroughly in tap water.
13. Counterstain with light green working solution for 30 to 45 seconds.
14. Dehydrate and clear through 95% ethyl alcohol, absolute ethyl alcohol, and xylene, 2 changes each, 2 minutes each.
15. Mount with resinous medium.

RESULTS (See Fig. 21-3, page 233).

Fungi .... sharply delineated in black
Mucin .... dark gray
Mycelia and hyphae .... gray rose
Background .... green

[a]If distilled water is not available, use sterile water or deionized water.

[b]Start checking for very light brown or tan color at 50 minutes, then at 55 minutes. Sections should be golden brown sometime between 55 to 60 minutes. Remove from oven immediately once the sections have started to turn a golden brown. Cool for several minutes before proceeding to the next step.

REFERENCE
Grocott RG. A stain for fungi in tissue sections and smears using Gomori methenamine silver nitrate technique. *Am J Clin Pathol.* 1955;25:975.

AFIP Laboratory Methods in Histotechnology

GROCOTT'S METHENAMINE SILVER
(Modified for microwave staining)

FIXATION: 10% buffered neutral formalin

SECTIONS: Paraffin, 4 to 6 micrometers

SOLUTIONS

10% CHROMIC ACID (Ch. 3)

5% SILVER NITRATE (Ch. 3)

2% SODIUM THIOSULFATE (Ch. 3)

3% METHENAMINE (Ch. 3)

5% BORAX (Ch. 3)

METHENAMINE-SILVER NITRATE STOCK SOLUTION
Silver nitrate, 5% solution ....5.0 ml
Methenamine, 3% solution .... 100.0 ml

METHENAMINE-SILVER NITRATE WORKING SOLUTION
Methenamine-silver nitrate solution, stock ....25.0 ml
Distilled water...25.0 ml
Borax, 5% solution ....2.0 ml
Prepare fresh prior to use. Do not use if cloudy.

1% SODIUM BISULFITE (Ch. 3)

1% GOLD CHLORIDE (Ch. 3)

0.2% LIGHT GREEN (Ch.3)

PROCEDURE
1. Deparaffinize and hydrate slides to distilled water.
2. Place in 10% chromic acid solution and microwave for 20 seconds at maximum power.
3. Let stand for 10 seconds in hot solution, then rinse in running tap water.
4. Place in 1% sodium bisulfite for 60 seconds.
5. Rinse in running tap water followed by 3 changes of distilled water.
6. Place slides in methenamine silver nitrate (working) solution and microwave for 20 seconds at maximum power.
7. Let slides stand in hot solution which has been placed in a beaker of water at

60°C for 30 or more seconds. The slides should remain until they are pale brown.

8. Rinse slides in 3 changes of distilled water.
9. Tone in 1% gold chloride for 10 seconds.
10. Rinse slides in distilled water.
11. Place in 2% sodium thiosulfate for 1 minute.
12. Wash in running tap water for 2 minutes.
13. Place in 0.2% light green for 30 seconds.
14. Rinse in distilled water.
15. Dehydrate, clear, and mount in resinous medium.

RESULTS

Fungi ....sharply delineated in black
Mucin ....taupe to dark gray
Inner parts of mycelia...old rose
Background ....pale green

REFERENCE

Brinn, NT. Rapid metallic histological staining using the microwave oven. *J Histotechnol.* 1983;6:125.

GRIDLEY'S METHOD FOR FUNGI

FIXATION: 10% buffered neutral formalin.

SECTIONS: Paraffin, 6 micrometers.

SOLUTIONS

4% CHROMIC ACID (CHROMIUM TRIOXIDE) SOLUTION (Ch. 3)

COLEMAN'S SCHIFF REAGENT (Ch. 18)

ALDEHYDE-FUCHSIN SOLUTION

Basic fuchsin	1.0 gm
Alcohol, ethyl 70%	200.0 ml
Hydrochloric acid, concentrated	2.0 ml
Paraldehyde	2.0 ml

Let stand at room temperature for 2 to 3 days.
Stain will be a deep purple color.

0.25% METANIL YELLOW SOLUTION

Metanil yellow	0.25 gm
Distilled water	100.0 ml
Acetic acid, glacial	0.25 ml

PROCEDURE
1. Deparaffinize and hydrate to distilled water.
2. Oxidize in 4% chromic acid solution for 1 hour.
3. Wash in running water for 5 minutes.
4. Place in Coleman's reagent for 15 minutes.[a]
5. Wash in running water for 15 minutes.[b]
6. Rinse in 70% alcohol, 2 changes.
7. Stain in aldehyde-fuchsin solution for 30 minutes.
8. Rinse off excess stain with 95% alcohol.
9. Rinse in distilled water.
10. Counterstain lightly with metanil yellow solution for 1 minute.
11. Rinse in distilled water.
12. Dehydrate and clear through 95% ethyl alcohol, absolute ethyl alcohol, and xylene, 2 changes each, 2 minutes each.
13. Mount with resinous medium.

RESULTS

Mycelia	deep purple
Conidia	deep rose to purple
Background	yellow
Elastic tissue and mucin	deep purple

ᵃDuring the staining process Coleman's reagent changes from colorless to a magenta color. This process has been shown to be enhanced by allowing the Coleman's reagent to come to room temperature before using or by placing the solution in a warm bath to reach and maintain a warm temperature.

ᵇRunning water may leach out the magenta color and cause the organisms to be understained. To prevent the loss of staining, slides are placed in warm tap water and allowed to stand. Slides are cleared with a rinse in tap water before starting the next step.

REFERENCE
Gridley MF. A stain for fungi in tissue sections. *Am J Clin Pathol.* 1953;23:303.

AFIP Laboratory Methods in Histotechnology

COATES MODIFIED FITE STAIN FOR NOCARDIA

FIXATIVE: 10% buffered neutral formalin or any well-fixed tissue.

SECTIONS: Paraffin, 4 to 6 micrometers.

SOLUTIONS

XYLENE-PEANUT OIL SOLUTION

Peanut oil ....1 part
Xylene ....2 parts

1% AQUEOUS SULFURIC ACID SOLUTION (Ch. 3)

ZIEHL-NEELSEN CARBOL-FUCHSIN SOLUTION

Phenol crystals, melted ....2.5 ml
Alcohol, absolute, ethyl ....5.0 ml
Basic fuchsin ....0.5 gm
Distilled water ....50.0 ml
Filter before use.

METHYLENE BLUE STOCK SOLUTION (Ch. 3)

METHYLENE BLUE WORKING SOLUTION (Ch. 3)

PROCEDURE
1. Deparaffinize with xylene-peanut oil solution, 2 changes, 12 minutes each.
2. Dip in xylene. Air-dry for 15 minutes.[a]
3. Stain in carbol-fuchsin solution for 10 minutes.[b]
4. Wash in tap water for 1 to 2 minutes.
5. Differentiate in 1% aqueous sulfuric acid solution for approximately 5 to 10 minutes. Agitate to remove background staining as quickly as possible; this will maintain the redness of the organism which is very fragile. The overall color will be purplish pink.
6. Wash in tap water.
7. Counterstain lightly with methylene blue working solution.
8. Rinse in tap water.
9. Blot and let stand for a few minutes to air-dry.[c]
10. Mount directly with resinous mounting medium.

RESULTS

Nocardia ....purplish red
Background ....light blue

aThe residual oil will leave a thin, oily film on the slides and tissue that helps to prevent shrinkage to the sections.

bThe time in the carbol-fuchsin solution is critical.

cFollowing air-drying of the slides, insert the optional quick dehydration and clearing with the use of 2 changes each of 95% and absolute ethyl alcohols and 2 changes of xylene. The advantages include a better differentiation of the counterstain and the removal of the residual oil. Do not let slides stand in alcohol, since alcohols decolorize the positive staining of the acid-fast organisms.

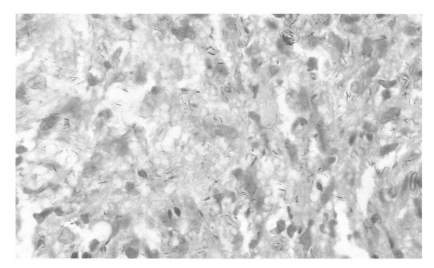

Fig. 21–1.
Fite stain.
Lepra bacilli in
skin.

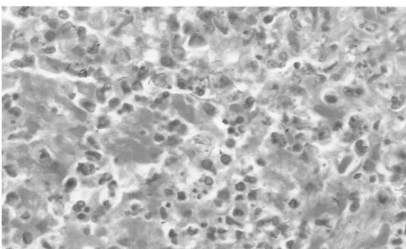

Fig. 21–2.
Ziehl-Neelsen
stain. Acid-fast
bacilli in lung.

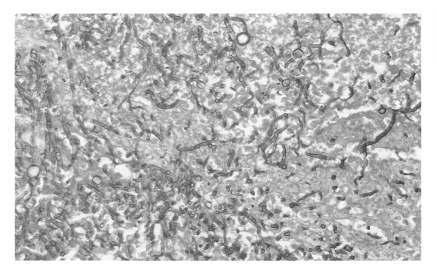

Fig. 21–3.
Grocott stain.
Aspergillus in
lung.

❖ CHAPTER 22

ENZYME HISTOCHEMISTRY

Diandrea Williams

A number of enzyme histochemical procedures are useful in the study of blood smears and other hematologic specimens. The blood films should be air-dried and, in general, not methanol fixed. Lymph nodes and splenic tissue can be fixed in buffered neutral formalin and cut as frozen sections. The search for hydrolytic enzyme activity in paraffin sections is generally unrewarding except for naphthol AS-D chloroacetate esterase (Leder procedure), which is well preserved. Decalcification, mercurial fixation or Bouin's fixation also make enzyme procedures unrewarding.

The following table shows the reactivities of hematologic cells with enzyme procedures.

Table 22-1

	Neutrophils	Monocytes & Histiocytes	Lymphocytes	Mast Cells	Eosinophils
Naphthol AS-D chloroacetate esterase (Leder)	+	-	-	+	-
Alphanaphthyl acetate esterase	+	+	T:+	-	-
Alphanaphthyl butyrate esterase	-	+	T:+	-	-
Alkaline phosphatase	+	-	B:+	-	-
Acid phosphatase	+	+	T:+	+	+
Myeloperoxidase	+	-	-	-	-

NAPHTHOL AS-D CHLOROACETATE ESTERASE (LEDER) PROCEDURE

FIXATION: 10% buffered neutral formalin.

SECTIONS: Paraffin, 6 micrometers; air dried blood smears and imprints.

SOLUTIONS

4% PARAROSANILINE STOCK SOLUTION

Pararosaniline hydrochloride .... 1.0 gm
Distilled water .... 20.0 ml
Hydrochloric acid, concentrated .... 5.0 ml

Gently warm solution to mix. Cool, filter, and store in refrigerator.

4% SODIUM NITRITE STOCK SOLUTION

Sodium nitrite .... 4.0 gm
Distilled water .... 100.0 ml

Store in refrigerator. Solution remains stable for 1 week.

SODIUM NITRITE PARAROSANILINE WORKING SOLUTION

Pararosaniline solution, 4% .... 2 drops
Sodium nitrite solution, 4% .... 2 drops

Prepare just before use. Let stand for 1 minute.

MICHAELIS VERONAL ACETATE BUFFER STOCK SOLUTION

Sodium acetate .... 9.7 gm
Sodium barbiturate .... 14.7 gm
Distilled water .... 500.0 ml

Store in refrigerator.

1 N HYDROCHLORIC ACID SOLUTION

Hydrochloric acid .... 85.0 ml
Distilled water .... 1000.0 ml

0.1N HYDROCHLORIC ACID SOLUTION

Hydrochloric acid, 1 N .... 10.0 ml
Distilled water .... 90.0 ml

MICHAELIS VERONAL ACETATE BUFFER WORKING SOLUTION

Michaelis veronal acetate buffer, stock solution ....45.0 ml
Hydrochloric acid, 0.1 N solution ....35.0 ml
Use 60.0 ml and reserve 20.0 ml.
Adjust pH to 6.3 using 1 N hydrochloric acid solution.

PARAROSANILINE/VERONAL ACETATE SOLUTION

Sodium nitrite/pararosaniline solution ....4 drops
Michaelis veronal acetate working buffer solution ....60.0 ml

ESTERASE SUBSTRATE SOLUTION

Naphthol AS-D chloroacetate ....20.0 mg
N-N dimethylformamide (DMF) ....2.0 ml
Prepare just before use.

PARAROSANILINE/VERONAL ACETATE ESTERASE SOLUTION

Pararosaniline veronal acetate solution, pH 6.3 ....60.0 ml
Esterase substrate solution ....2.0 ml
Mix well. Filter with fine grade paper just before using.

MAYER'S HEMATOXYLIN SOLUTION (Ch. 9)

PROCEDURE
1. Place deparaffinized and hydrated slides and blood smears in filtered pararo-saniline veronal acetate esterase solution for 30 to 120 minutes. Check slides microscopically every 30 minutes for the red-to-brown color indicating enzyme activity.
2. Rinse in distilled water for 2 minutes.
3. Counterstain in Mayer's hematoxylin solution for 5 minutes.
4. Rinse in distilled water.
5. Mount using aqueous medium.

RESULTS

Neutrophilic myeloid cells ....scarlet red
Tissue mast cells...scarlet red
Chediak-Higashi inclusions ....scarlet red
Nuclei ....blue

REFERENCES
Leder LD. The selective enzymochemical demonstration of neutrophillic myeloid cells and tissue mast cells in paraffin sections. *Klin Wochenschr.* 1964;42:533.

ALPHANAPHTHYL ACETATE ESTERASE

FIXATION: 10% buffered neutral formalin.

SECTIONS: Frozen and paraffin, 4 to 6 micrometers; smears and imprints.

SOLUTIONS

4% PARAROSANILINE STOCK SOLUTION

Pararosaniline hydrochloride ....1.0 gm
Distilled water ....20.0 ml
Hydrochloric acid, concentrated ....5.0 ml
Gently warm solution to mix. Cool, filter, and store in refrigerator.

4% SODIUM NITRITE STOCK SOLUTION

Sodium nitrite ....4.0 gm
Distilled water ....100.0 ml
Store in refrigerator. Solution remains stable for 1 week.

TRIS BUFFER SOLUTION, pH 7.6 (see Table 22-2)

SODIUM NITRITE/PARAROSANILINE SOLUTION

Sodium nitrite solution, 4% stock ....2 drops
Pararosaniline solution, 4% stock ....2 drops
Mix just before use. Then add:
Tris buffer solution, pH 7.6 ....50.0 ml
Mix thoroughly.

ESTERASE SUBSTRATE SOLUTION

Alphanaphthyl acetate ....0.02 gm
Ethylene glycol monoethyl ether ....2.0 ml
Prepare just before use.

ESTERASE SUBSTRATE/SODIUM NITRITE
PARAROSANILINE WORKING SOLUTION

Sodium nitrite/pararosaniline solution ....50.0 ml
Esterase substrate solution ....2.0 ml
Mix thoroughly.

MAYER'S HEMATOXYLIN SOLUTION (Ch. 9)

PROCEDURE
1. Place deparaffinized and hydrated sections, smears or imprints in the esterase substrate/sodium nitrite pararosaniline working solution at room temperature for 1-2 hours. Check sections every 15 to 30 minutes for the red-to-brown color that indicates enzyme activity.
2. Rinse thoroughly in distilled water for approximately 3 minutes.

3. Counterstain in Mayer's hematoxylin solution for 2-5 minutes.
4. Rinse well in distilled water.
5. Mount using aqueous mounting medium.

RESULTS

Cytoplasm of T-lymphocytes, neutrophils,
monocytes, and histiocytes .... red to brown

---

REFERENCES (For esterases):

Barka T, Andersen PJ. *Histochemistry Theory, Practice and Bibliography*. New York, NY: Hoeber; 1963.

Braunstein H. Esterase in leukocytes. *J Histochem Cytochem*. 1959;7:202.

Kulenkampff J, Janossy G, Graves MF. Acid esterase in human lymphoid cells and leukemic blasts: A marker for T-lymphocytes. *Br J Haematol*. 1977;36:231.

Li CY, Lam KW, Yam LT. Esterases in human leukocytes. *J Histochem Cytochem*. 1973;21 :1 .

Rindler-Ludwig R, Schmalzl F, Braunsteiner H. Esterses in human neutrophil granulocytes: Evidence for their protease nature. *Br J Haematol*. 1974;27:57.

ALPHANAPHTHYL BUTYRATE ESTERASE

FIXATION: Air-dried smears or imprints, 10% buffered neutral formalin.

SECTIONS: Frozen and paraffin, 4 to 8 micrometers; smears and imprints.

SOLUTIONS
4% PARAROSANILINE STOCK SOLUTION

Pararosaniline hydrochloride ....1.0 gm
Distilled water ....20.0 ml
Hydrochloric acid, concentrated ....5.0 ml
Gently warm solution to mix. Cool, filter, and store in refrigerator.

4% SODIUM NITRITE STOCK SOLUTION

Sodium nitrite ....4.0 gm
Distilled water ....100.0 ml
Store in refrigerator. Solution remains stable for 1 week.

PARAROSANILINE WORKING SOLUTION

Pararosaniline, 4% stock ....1.5 ml
Sodium nitrite, 4% stock ....1.5 ml
Combine, mix, and wait 5 minutes.

TRIS BUFFER SOLUTION pH 7.6 (see Table 22-2)

Prewarm to 37 °C.

SUBSTRATE WORKING SOLUTION

Tris buffer, pH 7.6 ....40.0 ml
Alphanaphthyl butyrate ....0.02 gm
Ethylene glycol monoethyl ether ....2.0 ml
Prepare just before use.

MAYER'S HEMATOXYLIN SOLUTION (Ch. 9)

PROCEDURE
1. Place deparaffinized, hydrated sections in distilled water, then in the substrate working solution. Place blood smears and touch imprints directly in substrate working solution. Check slides every 15 minutes for the red color to appear. Reaction usually takes 30 to 60 minutes.
2. Rinse in distilled water for 2-3 minutes. Air-dry for 15 minutes.
3. Counterstain in Mayer's hematoxylin for 2-5 minutes. Rinse in distilled water. Mount in aqueous medium.

RESULTS

Cytoplasm of monocytes and histiocytes ....red to brown
Golgi zone of T-lymphocytes ....red to brown
Cytoplasm of neutrophils and eosinophils ....no color

BURSTONE'S METHOD FOR ALKALINE PHOSPHATASE

FIXATION: Fresh frozen, 10% buffered neutral formalin, or formol-calcium.

SECTIONS: Frozen and paraffin, 4 to 8 micrometers; smears and imprints.

SOLUTIONS

NAPHTHOL AS-MX PHOSPHORIC ACID/(DMF)N,N DIMETHYLFORMAMIDE SOLUTION

Naphthol AS-MX phosphoric acid ....4.0 mg
N,N Dimethylformamide ....0.25 ml
Mix until completely dissolved.

TRIS BUFFER SOLUTION, pH 8.6 (see Table 22-2)

SUBSTRATE WORKING SOLUTION

Naphthol AS-MX phosphoric acid/DMF solution ....0.25 ml
Distilled water...25.0 ml
Tris buffer, pH 8.6 ....25.0 ml
Shake to mix thoroughly before adding:
Diazonium salt (red violet LB salt) ....30.0 mg

Filter. Insure that the ingredients are thoroughly mixed before filtering mixture into a Coplin jar. Use #12 Whatman filter paper. Solution should be clear and canary yellow.

MAYER'S HEMATOXYLIN SOLUTION (Ch. 9)

PROCEDURE
1. Place fresh frozen sections or deparaffinized and hydrated sections into substrate working solution for 5 to 30 minutes. Check slides every 5 or 10 minutes for the intense red color indicative of enzyme activity.
2. Rinse in distilled water.
3. Counterstain, if desired, in hematoxylin for 2 to 5 minutes.
4. Rinse in distilled water.
5. Mount with aqueous medium.

RESULTS
Neutrophils and B-lymphocytes ....intense red

REFERENCE

Burstone MS. Histochemical comparison of napthol AS phosphates for the demonstration of phosphatases. *J Natl Cancer Inst.* 1958;20:601.

BARKA'S METHOD FOR ACID PHOSPHATASE

FIXATION: 10% buffered neutral formalin; formol calcium.

SECTIONS: Frozen, 4 to 6 micrometers; air-dried smears and imprints.

SOLUTIONS

4% PARAROSANILINE STOCK SOLUTION

Pararosaniline hydrochloride ....1.0 gm
Distilled water...20.0 ml
Hydrochloric acid, concentrated.................................5.0 ml
Gently warm solution to mix. Cool, filter, and store in refrigerator.

4% SODIUM NITRITE STOCK SOLUTION

Sodium nitrite ....4.0 gm
Distilled water ....100.0 ml
Store in refrigerator. Solution remains stable for 1 week.

MICHAELIS VERONAL ACETATE BUFFER STOCK SOLUTION

Sodium acetate ....9.7 gm
Sodium barbiturate ....14.7 gm
Distilled water ....500.0 ml
Store in refrigerator.

SUBSTRATE WORKING SOLUTION

Solution A
Sodium alphanaphthol phosphate ....20.0 mg
Distilled water...13.0 ml
Michaelis veronal acetate buffer, stock ....5.0 ml

Solution B
Combine the following in a small test tube:
Pararosaniline stock solution ....0.8 ml
Sodium nitrite, 4% stock solution ....0.8 ml
Mix and let stand for 2 minutes.
Combine solutions A and B. Adjust pH to 6.5 using
  1 N sodium hydroxide.
Filter.

1 N SODIUM HYDROXIDE

Sodium hydroxide ....40.0 gm
Distilled water ....1000.0 ml

MAYER'S HEMATOXYLIN SOLUTION (Ch. 9)

PROCEDURE

1. Place air-dried frozen sections or blood smears into the substrate working solution at room temperature for 10 to 30 minutes.
2. Rinse in distilled water, 2 changes.
3. Counterstain in Mayer's hematoxylin solution for 2 to 5 minutes.
4. Rinse in distilled water.
5. Mount using aqueous medium.

RESULTS

Sites of enzyme activity .... red-to-brown precipitate

T-lymphocytes show positivity in the Golgi zone. Mast cells show weak positivity.

REFERENCE

Barka T, Anderson PJ. Histochemical methods for acid phosphatase using hexazonium pararosaniline as coupler. *J Histochem Cytochem.* 1962;10:741.

MYELOPEROXIDASE METHOD

FIXATION: 10% buffered neutral formalin (tissue), methanol (smears). Blood smears are fixed in methanol for 30 seconds, rinsed in distilled water, and then air-dried in the dark for 10 minutes.

SECTIONS: Paraffin, 6 micrometers; smears.

SOLUTIONS

3% HYDROGEN PEROXIDE SOLUTION (Ch. 3)

TRIS BUFFER SOLUTION, pH 6.3 (see Table 22-2)

PEROXIDASE INDICATOR REAGENT SOLUTION

p-Phenylenediamine ....25.0 mg
Catechol ....50.0 mg
Tris buffer, pH 6.3 ....50.0 ml

Preheat solution to 37°C for 5 minutes before adding 0.2 ml of 3% hydrogen peroxide solution.

1% SODIUM IODATE SOLUTION

Sodium iodate ....1.0 gm
Distilled water ....100.0 ml

ACID HEMATOXYLIN SOLUTION

Hematoxylin ....50.0 mg
Distilled water ....48.0 ml
Sodium iodate solution, 1% ....1.0 ml
Heat to boiling point. Cool and add:
Acetic acid, glacial ....2.0 ml

PROCEDURE

1. Incubate the deparaffinized and hydrated slides or blood smears in preheated (37°C) peroxidase indicator reagent solution, for 30 minutes.
2. Rinse in distilled water for 15 to 30 seconds.
3. Air-dry for 15 minutes.
4. Counterstain in acid hematoxylin solution for 10 minutes.
5. Rinse in distilled water for 15 to 30 seconds.
6. Air-dry for at least 15 minutes. Dip in xylene.
7. Mount using resinous medium.

RESULTS

Neutrophils and their precursors ....black to brown

Table 22- 2.

TRIS (HYDROXYMETHYL) AMINOMETHANE-MALEATE
(TRIS-MALEATE 0.05M)

BUFFER STOCK SOLUTIONS:
- A.   0.2M solution of tris-maleate (24.2 gm tris {hydroxymethyl}-amino-methane + 23.2 gm maleic acid, analytic grade or 19.6 gm maleic anhydride in 1000.0 ml distilled water).

- B.   0.2M sodium hydroxide (8.0 gm sodium hydroxide in 1000.0 ml distilled water.)

FORMULA FOR SOLUTIONS pH 5.2 to pH 8.6.

50.0 ml of A + X ml of B, then dilute to a final volume of 200.0 ml

pH	0.2M sodium hydroxide
5.2	7.0 ml
5.4	10.8 ml
5.6	15.5 ml
5.8	20.5 ml
6.0	26.0 ml
6.2	31.5 ml
6.4	37.0 ml
6.8	45.0 ml
7.0	48.0 ml
7.2	51.0 ml
7.4	54.0 ml
7.6	58.0 ml
7.8	63.5 ml
8.0	69.0 ml
8.2	75.0 ml
8.4	81.0 ml
8.6	86.5 ml

Adjust pH with Solution B or 1 N HCl.

CHAPTER 23

IMMUNOHISTOCHEMISTRY

Bob Mills

The increasing popularity and demand for immunohistochemical identification of specific substances have opened a new era for histopathology and histotechnology. Immunohistochemistry is the use of precisely selected antibodies to identify (mark) specific antigens. The tests are extremely sensitive and can usually detect very small amounts (e.g., nanograms or individual molecules) of a substance. There are numerous methods, reagents, and kits available. This discussion will be limited to the two most widely used methods: the Peroxidase Antiperoxidase (PAP) method and the Avidin Biotin Complex technique (ABC).

ANTIGENS AND ANTIBODIES

An antigen is a substance that when introduced into the body will stimulate an immune response (antibody production). In immunohistochemistry, an antigen is the substance that we are trying to demonstrate.

Antibodies are serum proteins (immunoglobulins) that are produced in response to specific substances (antigens). In the body their purpose is to counteract or neutralize the effect of the antigen. In the histology laboratory we "link" the antibody to the antigen in combination with a visual marker.

METHODS

Direct Method: A visual marker, either fluorescent or enzymatic, is chemically attached to the primary antibody. The primary antibody is the antibody that is directed against the antigen we want to demonstrate.

Indirect Method: The visual marker is attached to a secondary antibody. The tissue is first exposed to the primary antibody and then to the secondary antibody, which is directed against the primary antibody and will "link" with it.

Peroxidase Antiperoxidase (PAP) Method: This method uses a primary antibody, a secondary antibody, and an antibody that is produced against and linked with peroxidase enzyme (PAP complex). The secondary antibody is produced in a species different from the primary and PAP complex, and the primary antibody and PAP complex are produced from the same species. The secondary antibody therefore acts as a "bridge" or "link" antibody.

Avidin-Biotin Complex Method (ABC): This technique also uses three reagents: a primary antibody, a secondary antibody that is chemically bound to the vitamin biotin, and a complex of the glycoprotein avidin that is bound to biotin and peroxidase. Avidin has the ability to bind nonimmunologically four molecules of biotin. This strong affinity gives this method excellent sensitivity.

ANTIBODY SOLUTIONS

Antibody solutions are produced in several different forms: whole animal serum, IgG only, affinity purified reagent, and monoclonal antibodies. Whole serum is the least expensive solution to manufacture, but it also contains serum elements and antibodies other than the specific antibody. Serum IgG contains mostly antibodies, both specific and others. Affinity purified reagent contains only the specific antibodies that we want, but it may be more specific than needed and is expensive to make. Monoclonal antibody solutions are produced against a single characteristic antigenic determinant (epitope). B-lymphocytes are used for monoclonal antibody production, as they form an antibody against only one of an antigen's epitopes. A B-lymphocyte from an immunized animal is fused with a myeloma cell (a cancerous plasma cell) to form a hybrid cell. The hybrid cell can live longer than the B-lymphocyte and produces antibodies in culture. The hybrid cell is grown in tissue culture or in another animal. The antibodies are collected in either the supernate fluid of the culture or in the ascitic fluid of the animal.

SUBSTRATE REACTIONS

Enzymes are catalysts that act on a substrate to speed up its conversion to a product. The horseradish peroxidase (HRP) used in immunohistochemistry reacts with hydrogen peroxide, when in the presence of an electron donor, to form a colored molecule. The enzyme is not depleted and can continue to catalyze the reaction forming many colored molecules.

$$HRP + H_2O_2 + Electron\ Donor = Colored\ Molecule + H_2O + HRP$$

Examples of some of the available electron donors are: 3,3 Diaminobenzidine tetrahydrochloride (DAB) and 3-Amino-9-ethylcarbazole (AEC). DAB produces a brown end product and can be coverslipped with a resinous mounting medium. AEC produces a red end product and must be coverslipped with an aqueous medium. Both chemicals are considered possible carcinogens and should be used with great care.

NONSPECIFIC REACTIVITY

The primary or secondary antibodies can attach to highly charged tissue elements such as connective tissues, resulting in a positive staining reaction in sites other than those containing the primary antigen. These sites can be "filled," prior to staining, with proteins from nonimmune serum from the same animal species in which the secondary antibody is produced. This "filling" of the charged sites prevents the secondary antibody from attaching to the tissue and greatly reduces nonspecific reactivity.

A second source of nonspecific reactivity is called Endogenous Peroxidase Activity (EPA). Most tissues contain peroxidase, an enzyme that will react with the substrate chromagen described above in the same way that the reagent peroxidase that we attached to the antigen will react. This EPA is generally located in areas containing large numbers of blood cells. EPA can be irreversibly inhibited by treating the tissues with 3% hydrogen peroxide in methanol solution (10 ml 30% hydrogen peroxide solution + 90 ml absolute methanol) for 30 minutes prior to staining. The use of commercial 3% hydrogen peroxide solution, which is used for medicinal purposes, should be avoided since its use can cause tissue damage due to excessive bubbling and fizzing, especially on tissues containing a lot of blood.

FIXATION

Fresh 10% neutral buffered formalin (pH 7.0-7.6) is most likely the optimum fixative for immunohistochemistry. Tissue should be exposed to the fixative just long enough to achieve good preservation and morphology. Overfixation will cause the formation of excess aldehyde linkages that can block or mask antigen-binding sites and prevent the primary antibody from linking to the antigen. Tissues that have been overexposed to formalin can be digested with proteolytic enzymes such as trypsin or pepsin to "free" some of the binding sites.

PROCESSING

Routine paraffin processing procedures (Chapter 5) are adequate for immuno-histochemistry. Do not allow processing temperatures to exceed 60°C, since excess heat will destroy antigens and cellular morphology. It is especially important to use clean paraffin compounds and to be certain that all traces of paraffin and plastic additives are removed from the tissue during the deparaffinizing and hydration phase. Residual embedding media can cause nonspecific staining, incomplete staining, or suppress staining entirely.

SECTION ADHESIVES

Because of the numerous steps involved and the constant handling and especially when enzyme digestion is employed, sections often become dislodged from the slide and are subsequently lost. Several commercial slide adhesives are available to help prevent section loss. In the Tri-Service School at AFIP, we precoat our slides with a solution of casein glue such as Elmer's Glue-All (Borden, Inc. Columbus, Ohio) as follows:

PREPARATION OF SLIDES FOR IMMUNOHISTOCHEMISTRY
1. Place new, unused slides in a staining rack.
2. Agitate the slides in warm, soapy water for several minutes.
3. Wash all soap residue from the slides in a stream of running tap water, followed by several rinses in distilled water.
4. Rinse the slides in absolute ethyl alcohol and allow to air-dry.
5. Dip the usable portion of the slides (one at a time) in a freshly prepared 15% aqueous solution of casein glue. Wipe glue from the back of each slide with a clean, lint-free cloth.
6. Air-dry the slides in a dust-free area and store them in a standard slide box until needed.

SECTIONING (MICROTOMY)

Paraffin sections are cut at 5 µm and floated on a water bath containing distilled water that is heated to approximately 42°C. The selected sections are picked up with the precoated slides and dried horizontally (flat) on a 37°C warming tray overnight. Optionally, slides may be dried at 60°C for 30 minutes, but great care must be taken to insure that the slides are completely dry and not overheated.

CONCENTRATIONS

Valid staining of the target antigen can only be achieved if the antibody solutions are used at ideal concentrations. Correct antibody dilution is affected by every solution and procedure performed on the specimen: fixation, processing, buffer selection, staining temperature, humidity, and staining times, just to mention a few. The key to uniform, valid, and significant results is consistency during all phases of tissue handling and staining. When determining dilutions, times, temperatures, and processing schedules for your laboratory, change and evaluate only one thing at a time. Most commercially prepared kits come with antibody solutions that have been titered for optimal results under most conditions, providing that the manufacturer's directions are followed. Individually acquired solutions must be titered in your laboratory. Each antibody concentration must be determined in conjunction with the antibody with which it is intended to react. They are interdependent. The whole idea is to find the exact concentration of each antibody (primary, secondary, and PAP complex) that results in maximum specific staining with minimal or no background staining. This is no easy task, and a wide range of dilutions must be studied. Starting dilutions can often be obtained from the manufacturer. First determine the ideal concentration of primary and link (secondary) antibodies. Prepare accurate dilutions of the primary and link antibodies using very precise pipettes. Stain a slide from serial sections of a known positive tissue for every possible combination of dilutions, using a previously proven or manufacturer-recommended PAP complex concentration (Fig. 23-1). Be certain to include one slide incubated with normal (nonimmune) serum from the same species in which the primary antibody was created as a negative control (see "Controls" below).

Example: PAP Complex 1:100 (one part antibody + 99 parts buffer)

> Primary antibody: 1:10, 1:100, 1:500, 1:1000
> Secondary antibody: 1:10, 1:100, 1:500

Fig. 23-1

PRIMARY ANTIBODY DILUTIONS

LINK ANTIBODY DILUTIONS	NS	1:10	1:100	1:500	1:1000
NS	X	X			
1:10	X	X	X	X	X
1:100		X	X	X	X
1:500		X	X	X	X

It may be necessary to repeat the above procedure within a range of dilutions determined from these results, e.g., each solution at 1:100, 1:200, 1:300, 1:400, and 1:500. Once the concentration of primary and link antibodies is determined, set up a similar battery of slides using those concentrations and varying the concentration of the PAP complex.

CONTROLS

Both positive and negative controls are run with each set of slides during the staining process. For negative controls replace the primary antibody with normal nonimmune serum (NS) from the same animal species in which the primary antibody was produced. Positive controls are slides that are known to contain the target antigen, have shown strong positive results in the past, and are stained with the primary antibody. A total of four slides are stained for each patient tissue being studied. Table 23-1 shows the slides to be stained, the solution to use, and the expected results for a valid test.

Table 23-1

SLIDE	SOLUTION	RESULT
Patient tissue	Primary Antibody	?
Patient tissue	Normal Serum	Negative
Known positive	Primary Antibody	Positive
Known positive	Normal Serum	Negative

GENERAL LABORATORY TECHNIQUE

The solutions used in these techniques can be very expensive. To minimize solution waste, we stain our slides horizontally (flat) on elevated rods in a humidity chamber. Disposable laboratory droppers are used to drop just enough solution on the slide to cover the tissue. Laboratory wash bottles are used for rinsing the slides with phosphate-buffered saline solution. Use of a covered humidity chamber is important. The slides must not be allowed to dry during any step of the procedure.

The microwave oven may be used to reduce incubation times in all of the antibody and blocking serum steps listed below. An all plastic, vented humidity chamber must be used in the microwave oven. Incubation times will vary considerably depending on the power of the oven's magnetron and the type of humidity chamber used: a good starting point is to microwave for 7 to 10 seconds and let stand at room temperature for 5 minutes (whereas usual incubation is 30 minutes). The Mayer's hematoxylin nuclear stain (step 16 below) may be dropped directly on the slide and microwaved on high for 3 to 7 seconds instead of using the standard 5 minute staining time.

PEROXIDASE ANTIPEROXIDASE PROCEDURE (PAP)
(AFIP Tri-Service School Method)

FIXATION: 10% buffered neutral formalin.

SECTIONS: Paraffin, 5 micrometers, on glue-coated slides.

SOLUTIONS

3% HYDROGEN PEROXIDE METHANOL SOLUTION

Hydrogen peroxide, 30% solution ....3.0 ml
Methanol, absolute...97.0 ml

CAUTION: 30% Hydrogen peroxide is a very strong oxidizer. Avoid any contact with the skin or flammable materials. Use protective clothing.

NORMAL SERUM (Same species as bridge antibody)

NORMAL SERUM (Same species as primary antibody)

PRIMARY ANTIBODY SOLUTION

BRIDGE ANTIBODY SOLUTION

PEROXIDASE ANTIPEROXIDASE (PAP) COMPLEX SOLUTION

PHOSPHATE-BUFFERED SALINE (PBS), PH 7.0 TO 7.6 SOLUTION

Sodium phosphate, dibasic, anhydrous ....1.48 gm
Sodium phosphate, monobasic, anhydrous.............0.43 gm
Sodium chloride ....7.20 gm
Distilled water..1000.0 ml

DIAMINOBENZIDINE (DAB) SUBSTRATE SOLUTION

3'3' Diaminobenzidine ....42.0 gm
PBS ....100.0 ml
Hydrogen peroxide, 30% ....0.4 ml

Prepare just before use. CAUTION: 3'3' Diaminobenzidine (DAB) may be carcinogenic. Avoid breathing the dry powder and contact with the skin. Dispose of the DAB solution in plastic containers and add 10 ml of chlorine bleach for each 100.0 ml of DAB solution.

MAYER'S HEMATOXYLIN SOLUTION (Ch. 9)

TRYPSIN SOLUTION

Trypsin ....0.1 gm
Phosphate-buffered saline solution,
    (pH 7.0 to pH 7.6) ....100.0 ml

Prepare just before use.

PROCEDURE
1. Deparaffinize slides and hydrate to distilled water.
2. Block endogenous peroxidase activity in hydrogen peroxide methanol solution for 30 minutes.
3. Rinse in 2 changes of distilled water, 1 minute each.
4. Place in phosphate-buffered saline (PBS) for 2 minutes.
5. Optional: Digest slides in freshly prepared trypsin solution at 37°C for 3 to 10 minutes.
6. Rinse well with phosphate-buffered saline solution.
7. Place in normal serum from the same species in which the bridge antibody is produced for 30 minutes; drain, but do not rinse the slides.
8. Place in primary antibody for 30 minutes.
9. Rinse well with phosphate-buffered saline solution.
10. Place in secondary antibody for 30 minutes.
11. Rinse well with phosphate-buffered saline solution.
12. Place in peroxidase antiperoxidase (PAP) complex solution for 30 minutes.
13. Rinse well with phosphate-buffered saline solution.
14. Place in diaminobenzidine (DAB) substrate solution for 10 minutes.
15. Rinse well with phosphate-buffered saline solution, followed by a rinse with distilled water.
16. Counterstain with Mayer's hematoxylin solution for 5 minutes.
17. Wash in tepid water for 10 minutes.
18. Dehydrate and clear through 95% ethyl alcohol, absolute ethyl alcohol, and xylene, 2 changes each for 2 minutes each.
19. Mount with resinous medium.

AVIDIN BIOTIN COMPLEX (ABC) PROCEDURE
(AFIP Tri-Service School Method)

FIXATION: 10% buffered neutral formalin.

SECTIONS: Paraffin, 5 micrometers, on glue-coated slides.

SOLUTIONS

3% HYDROGEN PEROXIDE IN METHANOL

30% Hydrogen peroxide solution ....3.0 ml
Methanol, absolute ....97.0 ml

Prepare fresh daily. CAUTION: 30% hydrogen peroxide is a very strong oxidizer. Avoid any contact with the skin or flammable materials. Use protective clothing.

NORMAL SERUM (Same species as bridge antibody)

NORMAL SERUM (Same species as primary antibody)

PRIMARY ANTIBODY SOLUTION

BRIDGE (BIOTINALATED) ANTIBODY SOLUTION

ABC SOLUTION

PHOSPHATE-BUFFERED SALINE (PBS), PH 7.0 TO 7.6

Sodium phosphate dibasic, anhydrous ....1.48 gm
Sodium phosphate monobasic, anhydrous ....0.43 gm
Sodium chloride ....7.20 gm
Distilled water ....1000.0 ml

DIAMINOBENZIDINE (DAB) SUBSTRATE SOLUTION

3'3' Diaminobenzidine ....42.0 gm
PBS ....100.0 ml
Hydrogen peroxide, 30% ....0.4 ml

Prepare just before use. CAUTION: 3'3' Diaminobenzidine may be carcinogenic. Avoid breathing the dry powder and contact with the skin. Dispose of DAB solution in plastic containers and add 10 ml of chlorine bleach for each 100 ml of DAB solution.

MAYER'S HEMATOXYLIN SOLUTION (Ch. 9)

TRYPSIN SOLUTION

Trypsin ....0.1 gm
Phosphate-buffered saline solution.........................100.0 ml

Prepare just before use.

PROCEDURE

1. Deparaffinize slides and hydrate to distilled water.
2. Block endogenous peroxidase activity in 3% hydrogen peroxide methanol solution for 30 minutes.
3. Rinse in 2 changes of distilled water, 1 minute each.
4. Place in phosphate-buffered saline solution for 2 minutes.
5. Optional: Digest slides in freshly prepared trypsin solution at 37°C for 3 to 10 minutes.
6. Rinse well with phosphate-buffered saline solution.
7. Place in normal serum from the same species in which the bridge antibody is produced for 30 minutes; drain but do not rinse slides.
8. Place in primary antibody solution for 30 minutes.
9. Rinse well with phosphate-buffered saline solution.
10. Place in secondary biotinalated antibody solution for 30 minutes.
11. Rinse well with phosphate-buffered saline solution.
12. Place in avidin biotin complex solution for 30 minutes.
13. Rinse well with phosphate-buffered saline solution.
14. Place in diaminobenzidine substrate solution for 10 minutes.
15. Rinse well with phosphate-buffered saline solution, followed by a rinse with distilled water.
16. Stain with Mayer's hematoxylin solution for 5 minutes.
17. Wash in tepid water for 10 minutes.
18. Dehydrate and clear through 95% ethyl alcohol, absolute ethyl alcohol, and xylene, 2 changes each for 2 minutes each.
19. Mount with a resinous medium.

REFERENCE

Bourne J. *Handbook of Immunoperoxidase Staining Methods.* Santa Barbara, CA: Dako Corporation; 1983.

❖ CHAPTER 24

TRANSMISSION ELECTRON MICROSCOPY

Francine R. Hincherick

At the AFIP there are several transmission electron microscopes and as with other technical operations, the users have developed some variations in fixation, processing, embedding, sectioning, and staining techniques. The following is suggested as a basic method for the handling of specimens in the transmission electron microscopy laboratory.

FIXATION

Small, 1 mm³ pieces of tissues are fixed in 2.5%-3.0% glutaraldehyde in 0.2M Sorenson's sodium phosphate buffer. E.M. grade 8% glutaraldehyde is purchased in 10 ml vials and stored in the refrigerator (4°C - 5°C).

0.2 M SORENSON'S SODIUM PHOSPHATE BUFFER

Solution A (Stock)
        Sodium phosphate monobasic, monohydrate ....27.8 gm
        Distilled water (or sterile water) ....1000.0 ml

Solution B (Stock)
        Sodium phosphate dibasic, heptahydrate..............53.65 gm
        Distilled water (or sterile water) ....1000.0 ml

If sodium phosphate dibasic is not available, *anhydrous* sodium phosphate dibasic may be substituted. Use 28.49 gm in 1000 ml distilled water.

WORKING SODIUM PHOSPHATE BUFFER, pH 7.2

        Solution A, (Stock) ....28.0 ml
        Solution B, (Stock) ....72.0 ml
Combine.

FIXATIVE SOLUTION: WORKING GLUTARALDEHYDE

        Glutaraldehyde, 8% ....10.0 ml
        Working sodium phosphate buffer ....22.0 ml

Fix the 1 mm specimens for 2 hours, then transfer to working sodium phosphate buffer. Hold in refrigerator until ready for processing. The length of time in fixative may be varied from 2 hours to 24 hours and the temperature from refrigerated to room temperature.

POSTFIXATION
    All specimens are postfixed in 1% osmium tetroxide.

1% OSMIUM TETROXIDE

        Osmium tetroxide ....1.0 gm
        Working sodium phosphate buffer ....100.0 ml

    Prepare under hood. **Vapors are highly toxic.** Use protective gear.

PROCESSING

    Tissue specimens can be processed manually or automatically. For these two alternatives, the chemicals and reagents are the same. However, there are variations in time for each.
    All tissue fluids are processed manually.

SOLUTIONS

1% URANYL ACETATE SOLUTION

        Uranyl acetate ....1.0 gm
        Sterile water ....100.0 ml

    Store in brown bottle in refrigerator.

WORKING SODIUM PHOSPHATE BUFFER, pH 7.2 (see above)

EPOXY RESIN

        Epoxy resin (Effapoxy) ....48.0 ml
        DDSA, Dodecenyl ....18.0 ml
        NMA, Nadic methyl anhydride ....32.0 ml
        DMP 30, Tris-dimethyl amino-methyl phenol ....1.2 ml

    Mix epoxy resin and DMP 30 for 1 minute with magnetic stirrer. Add DDSA while stirring. Then add NMA while stirring. Mix for 30 minutes. Store working epoxy resin in disposable syringes, in the refrigerator. Solution remains usable for 3 days. Polymerize a block overnight, to insure adequate polymerization.

PROPYLENE OXIDE

25% STOCK ALBUMIN

    Solutions used in processing tissue fluids:
        Albumin ....25.0 gm
        Distilled water (or sterile water) ....100.0 ml

    For convenience and to save solution, the above may be prepared in a smaller quantity as 6.25 gm in 25.0 ml distilled water.

WORKING ALBUMIN SOLUTION

        Working sodium phosphate buffer solution ....10.0 ml
        Albumin, 25% stock solution ....5 drops

TRANSMISSION ELECTRON MICROSCOPY
PROCESSING SCHEDULE
MANUAL

1. Working phosphate buffer, 3 changes ....15 minutes each
2. Osmium tetroxide, 1.0% phosphate buffered ....1 hour
3. Distilled water, 4 changes ....15 minutes each
4. Uranyl acetate, 1% aqueous ....1 hour
5. 50% ethyl alcohol ....15 minutes
6. 75% ethyl alcohol ....15 minutes
7. 95% ethyl alcohol ....15 minutes
8. 100% (absolute) ethyl alcohol, 4 changes ....15 minutes each
9. Equal parts 100% ethyl alcohol and propylene oxide ....15 minutes
10. Propylene oxide, 4 changes ....15 minutes each
11. Equal parts propylene oxide and epoxy resin ....1 hour
12. Epoxy resin, 3 changes ....1 hour each
13. Epoxy resin ....2 hours
14. Embed

When using Osmium Tetroxide and Propylene Oxide **USE HOOD.**

TRANSMISSION ELECTRON MICROSCOPY
PROCESSING SCHEDULE
AUTOMATIC

1. Working phosphate buffer, 3 changes ....20 minutes each
2. Osmium tetroxide, 1.0% phosphate buffered ....1 hour
3. Distilled water, 3 changes ....30 minutes each
4. Uranyl acetate, 1% aqueous ....1 hour
5. 50% ethyl alcohol ....20 minutes
6. 70% ethyl alcohol ....20 minutes
7. 95% ethyl alcohol ....20 minutes
8. 100% ethyl alcohol, 2 changes ....30 minutes each
9. 100% ethyl alcohol...1 hour
10. Equal parts propylene oxide and 100% ethyl alcohol ....20 minutes
11. Propylene oxide, 2 changes ....20 minutes each
12. 3 parts propylene oxide and 1 part epoxy resin ....1 hour
13. Equal parts propylene oxide and epoxy resin ....1 hour
14. 1 part propylene oxide and 3 parts epoxy resin ....1 hour
15. Epoxy resin ....5 hours
16. Embed

MANUAL PROCESSING SCHEDULE FOR FLUIDS

1. Transfer fluid to a centrifuge tube.
2. Centrifuge, at 1500 rpm in a clinical centrifuge, for 8 minutes.
3. Syphon off supernatant fluid carefully.
4. Add working sodium phosphate buffer solution.
5. Centrifuge, at 1500 rpm, for 8 minutes.
6. Syphon off buffer from sediment. Repeat steps 4 through 6, 3 more times.
7. Resuspend the sediment in a few ml of buffer albumin mixture and place in a conical microfuge tube.
8. Centrifuge, at 1500 rpm, for 8 minutes.
9. Cut off the conical tip of the microfuge tube. Remove the cell block.
10. Place the cell blocks in working sodium phosphate buffer solution in a specimen jar.
11. Under a hood, pour off the sodium phosphate buffer solution and add sufficient quantity of 1% osmium tetroxide solution to cover cell blocks. Allow to remain for 1 hour.
12. Under a hood, decant the 1% osmium tetroxide solution. Fill the specimen jars containing the cell blocks with 3 changes of sterile water, 15 minutes each.
13. Place in 1% uranyl acetate solution for 1 hour.
14. Place in 50%, 70%, and 95% ethyl alcohol for 15 minutes each.
15. Place in 4 changes of absolute (100%) ethyl alcohol, 15 minutes each.
16. Equal parts absolute ethyl alcohol and propylene oxide, 15 minutes.
17. Place in propylene oxide, 3 changes, 15 minutes each.
18. Place in equal parts propylene oxide and epoxy resin for 1 hour.
19. Place in epoxy resin, 3 changes, 1 hour each.
20. Place in epoxy resin, 2 hours.
21. Embed.

EMBEDDING

The 1 mm^3 specimens are embedded in BEEM capsules. Routinely, size 00 is used. Before placing the processed specimens into the capsules, insert a typed identification number.

1. The capsules are place in embedding molds and filled with epoxy resin.
2. Specimens are placed at the tip.
3. Orientation is checked with a stereoscope.
4. Close the caps.
5. Place the closed capsules in embedding molds, in a 72°C oven to polymerize, for 24 to 48 hours.
6. When polymerization is complete, remove the epoxy blocks with a BEEM press.
7. Store embedded specimens in pill-boxes with all identifying information written clearly on the outside of the box.

AFIP Laboratory Methods in Histotechnology

THICK SECTIONING

To identify areas of interest, it is necessary to take 0.5 -1 micrometer thick sections which, when stained, are examined under the light microscope. Those sections which demonstrate "areas of interest" will be thin sectioned later.

1. Place the block in the block holder.
2. With the aid of a stereoscope (or on an ultramicrotome) gradually trim the epoxy from the surface of the block. Use a single edge razor blade. This process is called "rough trimming".
3. Continue trimming until the tissue is exposed and a smooth surface is achieved. An exposed square surface of 0.5 mm to 1 mm is ideal.
4. To facilitate sectioning, the block face is trimmed into a trapezoid shape, with top and bottom sides parallel.
5. Insert the block into the ultramicrotome.
6. Using a glass knife, fine trim the surface of the block to a shiny lustre.
7. Sections are collected in a trough filled with distilled water, which is level with the knife edge.
8. Retrieve the sections with an applicator stick and place on a drop of water on a premarked slide.
9. Dry on a hot plate set for "medium heat" for 30 minutes.
10. Cool and then stain with toluidine blue.

THICK SECTION STAINING

SOLUTIONS

1% SODIUM BORATE

Sodium borate .... 1.0 gm
Distilled water .... 100 0 ml

2% TOLUIDINE BLUE O IN SODIUM BORATE

Toluidine blue O .... 2.0 gm
Sodium borate, 1% .... 100.0 ml

STAINING PROCEDURE

1. Flood sections with the toluidine blue solution.
2. Place slides on a hot plate for approximately 1 minute. Edges of the stain will have a sheen.
3. Rinse in sterile water.
4. Air dry completely.
5. Coverslip with resinous medium.

   The pathologist reviews the slides and indicates the areas of interest for thin sectioning. A drawing of the "trapezoid" and specific markings aid the technologists in thin sectioning.

THIN SECTIONING

The block selected for "thins" is placed in the block holder and with the aid of the stereoscope is trimmed smaller for thin sections. The trapezoid shape is retained and the pathologist's drawing is used to eliminate unwanted areas.

1. Place trimmed block in the ultramicrotome
2. Using a diamond or glass knife, cut the thin sections at the desired thickness.
3. Collect the thin sections in a trough.
4. Examine the thin sections using the stereoscope binoculars. Raise or lower to observe the "colors" of the sections. These so called "interference colors" should be in the gray to gold range. Silver to gray sections are approximately 500-600 Ångstroms. Silver to gold sections are approximately 700-900 Ångstroms.
5. Pick up sections by inserting into the trough, a 200 mesh grid held with forceps. The grid is brought under the sections and then raised.
6. Drain the grid on filter paper.
7. Store grids in Petri dishes, on filter paper labeled with the identification numbers.

Sections should be thin enough for adequate beam penetration to achieve good resolution. High quality thin sections will have no chatter, knife lines, cracks, folds, or contamination.

MANUAL GRID STAINING

SOLUTIONS

35% METHANOL
Methanol .... 35.0 ml
Sterile water .... 65.0 ml

4% URANYL ACETATE IN METHANOL
Uranyl acetate .... 4.0 gm
Methanol, 35% .... 100.0 ml

1N SODIUM HYDROXIDE (see Ch. 3)

LEAD CITRATE
Lead nitrate .... 1.33 gm
Sodium citrate .... 1.76 gm
Sterile water .... 30.00 ml

Shake the above ingredients in a 50 ml flask for 20 minutes. Add 8 ml of 1 N sodium hydroxide. Dilute to 50 ml with sterile water. Mix by inversion. The solution is ready for use when completely clear.

PROCEDURE
1. Place 5 ml of uranyl acetate solution and 5 ml of lead citrate solution in *separate* screw top vials, Falcon tubes 13 X 100 mm, then centrifuge *each* at high speed 1500 rpm for 5 minutes.
2. Prepare two Petri dishes, lining each with a square of dental wax . Label #1 and #2.
3. Place several drops of centrifuged uranyl acetate on wax in Petri dish #1, one

drop of uranyl acetate for each grid to be stained. Keep dishes covered before and during staining.

4. Place sodium hydroxide pellets under wax in Petri dish #2.
5. Place several drops of lead citrate on wax, one drop for each grid to be stained.
6. Transfer grids, specimen side down, with the aid of fine forceps, onto the uranyl acetate drops in Petri dish #1. Stain in covered dish for 10 minutes.
7. Remove grids with fine forceps.
8. Rinse well with sterile water using a syringe.
9. Dry grids on clean filter paper or lens paper.
10. Stain in lead citrate, Petri dish #2, for 5 minutes.
11. Remove grids with fine forceps.
12. Rinse well with sterile water using a syringe.
13. Dry grids on clean filter paper or lens paper.

Index

B

C

NOTES